Building Relationships and Communicating with Young Children

Why is it important for social workers to form meaningful relationships with young children on their caseloads? And how can social workers develop these relationships?

This book provides a timely, invaluable resource and practical guide for social work students specializing in family and child care and for practitioners who have young children on their caseloads. Packed with real-life examples of in-depth interviews conducted with young children known to social services, it outlines what can be done to improve practice in this challenging and demanding area.

Building Relationships and Communicating with Young Children is the first book to bring to life the perspectives of young children and to highlight their competency within the interview process. It:

- explores the key ingredients required by social workers to establish, maintain, nurture and value their relationships with young children;
- highlights what young children, within the context of meaningful relationships with social workers, can tell us about their circumstances, their perspectives, their feelings and their views;
- uses real-life case examples to identify best practice guidelines including methods and techniques for social workers to build meaningful relationships with young children;
- makes recommendations regarding how best to positively engage and work with young children.

Written by a social worker and university lecturer with 16 years' experience of working in the field of child protection, this textbook is full of case studies and practical advice about how to form relationships with young children known to social services, the most appropriate methods to use and how to represent their perspectives. It is essential reading for all social work students as well as social work practitioners and other social- and health-care professionals.

Karen Winter is Lecturer in Social Work at Queen's University Belfast, UK. A qualified social worker for 16 years, she has worked in family and child care and as a Guardian ad Litem.

Building Relationships and Communicating with Young Children

A practical guide for social workers

Karen Winter

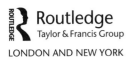

Routledge
Taylor & Francis Group

LONDON AND NEW YORK

First published 2011
by Routledge
2 Park Square, Milton Park, Abingdon, Oxon, OX14 4RN

Simultaneously published in the USA and Canada
by Routledge
270 Madison Avenue, New York, NY 10016

Routledge is an imprint of the Taylor & Francis Group, an informa business

© 2011 Karen Winter

Typeset in Sabon by
Pindar NZ, Auckland, New Zealand
Printed and bound in Great Britain by
TJ International Ltd, Padstow, Cornwall

British Library Cataloguing in Publication Data
A catalogue record for this book is available from the British Library

Library of Congress Cataloging-in-Publication Data
Winter, Karen.
Building relationships and communicating with young children: a practical guide for social workers / Karen Winter.
   p. cm.
  1. Social work with children. 2. Interpersonal relations. 3. Interpersonal communication. I. Title.
  HV713.W56 2011
  362.7—dc22   2010022489

ISBN13: 978-0-415-56267-6 (hbk)
ISBN13: 978-0-415-56268-3 (pbk)
ISBN13: 978-0-203-83672-9 (ebk)

Contents

Illustrations

Figures

Tables

Acknowledgements

There are a number of people I would like to thank who have helped me write this book. First and foremost I would like to thank the young children, parents and social workers for their invaluable time and willingness to participate in the research that is discussed in this book. It is through their perspectives that we gain so much insight and a desire to change things for the better.

I am also indebted to Nicola Carr and Caroline Leeson who offered encouragement and/or kindly agreed to read various parts of the book in draft and whose comments I have found extremely useful. A very special thank you is also due to Priscilla Alderson who did all this and so much more. Her unwavering commitment to the issue of young children's rights is truly inspiring.

Finally, and as always, I am most indebted to my partner, Paul Connolly. He has spent so much time reading through and commenting on the whole of the book and, in so doing, has helped me to develop and refine my ideas. He is a very wise counsel as well as my best friend.

This book is dedicated to my children – Mary (aged 10), Orla (aged 9) and Rory (aged 8) – who remind me every day of the importance of relationships.

Abbreviations

ANV	A National Voice
CAF	Common Assessment Framework
CRAE	Children's Rights Alliance for England
CWDC	Children's Workforce Development Council
CYPU	Children and Young People's Unit (England)
DH	Department of Health (England)
DHSS	Department of Health and Social Security (England)
DHSSPSNI	Department of Health, Social Services and Public Safety Northern Ireland
DCSF	Department for Children, Schools and Families (England)
DfES	Department for Education and Skills (England)
ECM	*Every Child Matters*
GIRFEC	Getting it Right for Every Child (Scotland)
GSCC	General Social Care Council (England)
HC CSF	House of Commons Children, Schools and Families Select Committee
HMSO	Her Majesty's Stationery Office
LAC	looked-after children
LSCB	Local Safeguarding Children Board
NCB	National Children's Bureau
NICCY	Northern Ireland Commissioner for Children and Young People
NISCC	Northern Ireland Social Care Council
SACR	Scottish Alliance for Children's Rights
SCIE	Social Care Institute for Excellence
SWTF	Social Work Task Force (England)
UN	United Nations
UNCRC	United Nations Convention on the Rights of the Child
UNOCINI	Understanding the Needs of Children in Northern Ireland
VCC/NCB	Voice for the Child in Care/National Children's Bureau
WMTD	What Makes the Difference project

Introduction

The legislation makes it plain that it is the well being of the child which should be the focus of all of the work by all of the agencies. That is clear in law. Too often agencies' attention is diverted onto the adult agenda [. . .] and too often all of the professions have a tendency to be too easily reassured, too optimistic and they don't think how vulnerable a child can be in those particular circumstances. And if [social workers] kept their attention on what it is like in the day of a child, what it feels like to be a child in those circumstances [then that] would influence the way in which they react.

(Lord Laming 2008)

Every two or three years social work with young children hits the national headlines and leads to much soul-searching by social workers, managers and policy makers. Each time it is usually precipitated by a critical incident involving the death of a young child known to social services. The latest, at the time of writing this book, involves a 17-month-old boy described initially by the media as 'Baby P' and who was subsequently named as Peter Connelly. He was known to social services and yet still met a horrific death due to neglect and abuse. His death led to an independent review by Lord Laming about the state of child protection in England (Laming 2009). As noted above in a BBC interview with Lord Laming, he concluded in his review that the problems in the case of Peter Connelly were not so much the absence of policies and procedures, which he determined were essentially sound, but were more about organizational deficits and the absence of good practice by professionals at the grass-roots level to implement those policies and procedures.

Peter Connelly died in the home of his mother and stepfather in the London Borough of Haringey on 3 August 2007. The post-mortem revealed that he had suffered a catalogue of appalling injuries at the hands of his carers in the preceding weeks and months including, at the time of his death, eight broken ribs and a broken back, bruises, cuts and lacerations to his head and body, missing fingernails and a missing front tooth which had been knocked out and was subsequently found lodged in his colon. When Peter's case came to the attention of the media in 2008 it caused a huge public outcry. Over a million people signed a petition organized by *The Sun* newspaper demanding that the professionals involved in the case be held to account for their failure to safeguard Peter's welfare. People were shocked because of Peter's injuries, his young age and, most significantly, the fact that his name was on the child protection register and social workers and other professionals had been regularly visiting him. And yet, despite all of this activity, not one professional had a close enough relationship with him to piece together the different facets of his chronically abusive experiences, to make sense of his deteriorating well-being, to establish his own views and feelings, or to act decisively on his behalf.

One could be forgiven for thinking that such an appalling catalogue of events as evident in the case of Peter Connelly is unique. Sadly, however, cases such as this that point to organizational deficits and the failure of social workers developing meaningful relationships with children in their care are not new but occur with depressing frequency. For as long as there have been inquiries into the care of children by social services there have been expressions of concern about poor-quality social worker relationships with young children. For example, it was back in 1945 that the first public inquiry of its kind was held following the death of Dennis O'Neill aged 12 years from horrific injuries sustained as a result of the abuse and neglect meted out at the hands of his foster carers. The inquiry noted the part played by infrequent social worker visits, the lack of personal, direct individual social worker engagement with Dennis and the failure of the social worker to act decisively when concerns were noted (Home Department 1945). Since then there have been over 70 similar public inquiries. The findings of some of these, particularly the deaths of Maria Colwell (DHSS 1974), Jasmine Beckford (London Borough of Brent 1985), Kimberley Carlisle (London Borough of Greenwich 1987), Tyra Henry (London Borough of Lambeth 1987) and Victoria Climbié (Laming 2003), bear striking similarity to the findings of the 1945 inquiry led by Sir Monckton and to the most recent reports into the death of Peter Connelly (Haringey LSCB 2009; Laming 2009).

While it is true to say, as Lord Laming (2009) notes, that improvements have been made, it is also true to say that concerns remain. As Laming points out, while the legislative frameworks and policies are now in place there remain significant concerns regarding their implementation. In particular, there are concerns about the capacity and the competence of the social work workforce to carry out the complex work demanded in the field of child protection, particularly in terms of building relationships and communicating effectively with young children. It is with this in mind that the purpose of this book is to highlight the importance of social workers' positive relationships with young children, how these can be achieved and what improvements can be made. It is hoped that this book, with its focus on real-life case examples and practice, will help to develop social workers who can be relied on to defend and champion the interests, rights and welfare of young children.

One of the motivations for me writing this book arises from my own experiences as a social worker, a team manager and most recently a Guardian ad Litem working in the area of child protection with children and families for over 16 years. During this time I have found that the very aspect of the job that motivated me to become a social worker – building relationships with children – was the one thing I sometimes found the most difficult to achieve. These relational aspects of my work, often viewed as a luxury rather than as essential, took a back seat because of all the other core demands of the job including form-filling, attendance at court hearings and other statutory meetings.

The routine lack of relationships developed by social workers with young children in their day-to-day practice was only really brought home to me when I began working as a Guardian ad Litem. A Guardian ad Litem is a qualified social worker appointed by the courts to represent children in court proceedings in private matters (divorce and separation) and public matters (care proceedings instigated by local authorities/trusts).

For the children I represented, it was part of my role to read all case material held on them. I noted that on numerous forms used for the 'looked-after' child review meetings (also called LAC or 'child in care' review meetings), it was stated of the younger children that they were 'unable to express their wishes and feelings'. However, I knew this was wrong. The case of one young boy, aged 8 years, proved very poignant and cathartic in this respect. Carter (I will not be using any real names) was referred to court because of chronic failure to thrive. There were unresolved and heated exchanges between his parents and other professionals about how his current and future needs should be met. In all this, he was relegated to being a silent observer to these discussions in which the many strong-minded adults in his life were locked in battle regarding who knew him best and what should happen to him.

As his newly appointed Guardian ad Litem, I met him in the home of his foster carer. He was sitting on the floor playing with Lego. I sat on the floor with him and we played together. He said nothing but just listened. I told him that it was my job to find out what it was like to be him and that I needed his help to do this. After more silent play, he picked up a Lego man and hid it behind a Lego wall so I could no longer see the figure. He then looked at me and simply said, 'I feel like I'm invisible'. We looked at each other in silence for a while. He then recounted examples of why he felt like this. A connection was formed that went way beyond the encounter itself because it reminded me of many other similar previous professional experiences. My meeting with Carter became a critical incident in my own career as it highlighted the broader position of young children and how they tend to be routinely ignored.

This book is about putting things right. It is about stressing the importance of the social worker–child relationship and the knowledge, skills and values required by social workers to build those relationships and to communicate meaningfully and effectively with young children. It is also about highlighting, through real-life case studies, the competence and capacities of young children to engage in relationships with adults. This book is based on both my substantial professional experience and the findings of original research that I have undertaken consisting of detailed case studies of ten families and involving in-depth interviews with 39 social workers, parents and young children (aged 4–7 years). The children were selected from those previously known to me in a professional capacity when I was their Guardian ad Litem but where that relationship had ended and the case had been closed. The research involved in-depth interviews with the children, their parents and social workers regarding young children's rights to participate in all matters affecting them as defined within the context of the United Nations Convention on the Rights of the Child (UN 1989). The interviews with the children involved the use of innovative participatory methods to facilitate exploration and expression of their views and feelings regarding their lives at home, their removal into care and their care experiences with a particular focus on their involvement in decision-making. As will be seen in the chapters to follow, the findings of the research revealed the detailed insights and deeply held feelings of young children regarding these aspects of their lives and also their competence, within the context of a trusting relationship, to express their views.

It is with these experiences in mind that this book seeks to highlight the value of social workers developing meaningful relationships with young children in terms of giving them the time and space to share their perspectives and for these to be taken seriously. This book makes public the hitherto often overlooked perspectives and views of this group of children. In doing so it demonstrates, through the voices of the children themselves, what their experiences are, their levels of competence and what can be achieved in terms of building meaningful relationships and communicating effectively with young children.

The book begins, in Chapter One, by setting the scene through a detailed analysis of the findings from official inquiry reports with the aim of understanding, in more detail, the nature of the failings of social workers' relationships with young children. The chapter shows that the inquiry reports reveal gaps in practice that are repeated by different social workers at different times and with different families. This suggests that these gaps reflect something endemic in relation to current social work practice and that the nature and quality of social worker relationships with young children requires detailed consideration. With these findings from the inquiry reports as the baseline, Chapter Two then considers in more detail the importance of relationships between children and their social workers and considers this from the perspectives of both the social workers and the children. The chapter highlights that even though there is widespread acceptance that relationships are important, and that there have been significant changes in legislation and policy that seek to reprioritize the centrality of relationships, social work practice with young children still causes concern.

Chapter Three then begins to explore some of the broader factors that are at the heart of these concerns by focusing on the organizational norms of the social work profession. It highlights that social work practice embodies broader organizational norms that tend to create barriers to building relationships and communicating with young children. Examples are provided through interviews with social workers conducted as part of my research. The chapter suggests that a new practice framework is required that is child rights-based, that can be adopted at both the organizational and individual levels and that seeks to support and encourage the development of a relationship-based practice with young children. Chapter Four then moves on to outline the specific details of this practice framework. The chapter suggests that a more sociologically informed framework, combined with a child rights perspective, would help in terms of building relationships. This new framework combines alternative ways of understanding young children alongside a concern for their rights. The chapter concludes by stressing that it is only when the frameworks to help build relationships are in place that meaningful communication between social workers and children is most likely to occur.

With the practice framework established, attention is turned in the next two chapters to implementing it into practice. Chapter Five focuses specifically on social workers' communication skills with young children. Using detailed case examples, drawn from my research, the chapter illustrates the skills required for effective communication at the different stages of the interview process. Building upon this Chapter Six then provides, with reference again to examples from my research, a detailed consideration of the methods used to facilitate communication with young children. The chapter highlights the importance of social workers paying attention to power imbalances, boundaries and ethical issues when using these methods and of respecting the choices, individuality, agency and views of the young children as they explore their perspectives.

Chapter Seven illustrates the many skills and methods outlined in previous chapters by showing them in action through the use of real-life in-depth case studies involving young children between the ages of 4 and 7. Alongside the skills of the social worker, the chapter also considers the contribution of children to the communication process through the use of various methods. The chapter draws out the various complex and deeply held views and feelings of young children and practical ways of responding to these.

The book draws to a close in Chapter Eight by drawing out and summarizing the key messages arising from the earlier chapters and suggesting recommendations for changes in practice at the levels of individual social workers, team managers and those responsible for resource allocation in order to help safeguard the lives and well-being of young children by prioritizing the development of meaningful relationships between them and social workers.

1   Setting the scene

Summary of chapter content

This chapter focuses on concerns about social worker relationships with young children through an overview of the findings of some of the key child abuse inquiries and serious case reviews that have taken place in the UK over the last 60 years. The chapter shows that strikingly similar difficulties have emerged at different times, in different places and with different children. These difficulties have included infrequent and inconsistent visits, visits that focus on the parents and the lack of direct personal communication by the social worker with the children. The chapter concludes by arguing that there is a need for practitioners to refocus on the importance and value of effective relationships with young children.

Introduction

Within the UK, the reports of over 70 child abuse public inquiries have been published since 1945 (Corby *et al.* 1998). Within the social work profession there have been mixed reactions to these. For example, Corby (2000: 220) has highlighted that 'there is considerable disagreement among social work professionals, trainers and educators about the value of utilizing inquiry reports in [. . .] teaching [and training]'. He has argued this is because some professionals have felt that, following public inquiries, a number of negative consequences tend to follow for the profession including an increased emphasis on bureaucracy and managerialism. Others have thought that there is an overemphasis on the 'individual pathology' of abusers as opposed to social and structural failings (Corby 2000: 220). Still others have felt that inquiry reports focus on individual practice in a vacuum and do not relate failings in practice to wider organizational and structural issues such as the lack of resources. While understanding these concerns, this chapter takes the view that engaging with and understanding the findings of child abuse inquiries is a critical part of social workers' reflection and learning. As Corby has argued, inquiries 'provide detailed accounts of professional involvement in child abuse cases of a kind which is rare elsewhere in social work literature: in effect, detailed 'real-life' case scenarios' (Corby 2000: 220). Furthermore, it is possible to see the huge influence that inquiries have on social work legislation, policy and practice. Most recently this has involved the social work reforms that have followed the Laming reports (2003, 2009), which investigated the circumstances surrounding the deaths of Victoria Climbié and Peter Connelly (see DCSF 2009c, 2009d; DH and DCSF 2009).

The focus for this chapter is not so much on the myriad of recommendations that have flowed from each of the inquiry reports but rather on the reported descriptions about the quality and nature of the social workers' relationships with the children involved. This approach does risk perpetuating the view that it is individual social workers who are to be named, blamed and shamed. However, it is argued that individual social work practice is a product of its broader context while also being able to shape that context. What this means is that while individual social workers need to take responsibility for their own practice, it is also important to recognize that their assumptions and working practices are also an embodiment of the norms and expectations of their organization. Within this context, it is therefore not acceptable simply to place the blame for failings squarely onto the shoulders of individuals. However, neither is it acceptable to lay blame solely at the level of the organization (the local authority, the trust, the team and the office). This is because social workers are free, within the constraints of the organization, to reflect on their assumptions and practices, to adapt them and thus to play some role, however limited, in helping to reshape and redefine their broader organizational context.

In considering some of the key findings that have emerged from the official inquiry reports, the chapter provides a chronological account of some of the major and most well-known inquiries that have taken place in each decade since the 1940s and uses these to draw out the key lessons for practitioners in their relationships with young children. I make no apologies for reviewing the findings in this way. Inquiries deal with the lives of real children and detail some of the horrific consequences they have faced when adults have failed to develop meaningful relationships with them. Moreover, in describing some of the case details contained in a number of reports and considering them side by side in this way, the key messages for social workers become abundantly clear.

The Monckton Report into the death of Dennis O'Neill (Home Department 1945)

> The 'fit person', local authority or individual, must care for the children as his own: the relation is a personal one. The duty must neither be evaded nor scamped.
>
> (Home Department 1945: 15, para. 46)

These were the words of Sir Monckton in his inquiry report (Home Department 1945) into the death of Dennis O'Neill, a 12-year-old boy who was known to social services and who died following sustained neglect and physical abuse at the hands of his foster carers. The case was the first of its kind to highlight the vulnerabilities of children placed in alternative care without adequate social worker supervision and support. In November 1939, Dennis and his three siblings (Terence, Freddie and Rosina) were removed from their parents' home and were, under the then existing legal provisions, taken to a place of safety following long-standing neglect and abuse. They remained under this arrangement until the end of May 1940 when a magistrate's court decided that Rosina could live with her maternal grandmother and the three boys should be committed to the care of Newport Council.

Newport Council was required to board out the children with suitable foster-parents. Between 30 May 1940 and 28 June 1944 the three brothers were boarded out with two sets of foster carers. Then, on 28 June 1944, Dennis was boarded out with Mr and Mrs

Gough who lived at Bank Farm in Shropshire. Terence joined him a week later, whereas Freddie was placed with other foster carers nearby. Six months later, on 9 January 1945, Dennis died having endured sustained abuse and neglect in the foster home. The cause of death was noted as 'acute cardiac failure following violence applied to the front of the chest and the back while in a state of under-nourishment' (Home Department 1945: 3, para. 3). Dennis had been beaten on the chest and back with a stick used by his foster-father. At the post-mortem he was noted to have septic ulcers on his feet and severely chapped legs. It was later revealed that the night before his death Dennis had been stripped naked, tied to a bench and beaten about the legs with a stick until his legs were blue and swollen and he could no longer stand. He was then locked in a small cupboard area. The testimony of his brother, Terence O'Neill, at the court proceedings of Mr and Mrs Gough, and his recently published book about their experiences (O'Neill 2010), reveal a catalogue of terrifying and appalling abuse.

In trying to understand how Dennis could have been so catastrophically let down, Sir Monckton's official inquiry concluded that Dennis's death could be in part attributed to the social worker's lack of personal relationship with him. Sir Monckton outlined three concerns in this regard: infrequent visits by the social worker to the new place-ment; lack of personal, direct individual engagement with Dennis by the social worker when visits did occur; and failure of the social worker to act decisively when concerns were noted.

On the third point, Sir Monckton said the social worker, on a home visit, saw that

> Dennis looked ill and frightened, answered questions extremely nervously and did not look up when answering [and that very] early in the interview she reached the conclusion that the children ought to be immediately removed.
>
> (Home Department 1945: 14, para. 38)

Although this was an unequivocal opinion, it was not followed up by decisive action. Rather than act on these observations and 'take the children away there and then' (Home Department 1945: 14, para. 41) Dennis and Terence were left in their placement while a request for a placement move was processed internally. During the time the request was being processed Dennis died. In summing up, Sir Monckton stated,

> I cannot escape the conclusion that there was in neither [local] authority a sufficient realisation of the direct and personal nature of the relationship between a super-vising authority and boarded-out children, that there was too great a readiness to assume that all was well without making sure.
>
> (Home Department 1945: 17, para. 50)

In highlighting the failures, Sir Monckton compared the social worker–child relationship with the parent–child relationship. He ascribed the former the same significance as the latter, arguing that both should be underpinned by the same qualities and character-istics. In effect what he was saying was that we, as social workers, need to think, feel, communicate, invest and act as if the children on our caseloads are our own. What is it in positive parent–child relationships that Sir Monckton was appealing to?

In reading the inquiry report, these characteristics seem to include: the nature of the parent–child relationship (based on responsibilities carried out within the context of a long-term, warm and consistent relationship); parenting skills (advocacy, insight, responsiveness, ability to offer 'care'); and the right conditions (resources and time). Sir Monckton's views on the relationships among the state, parenthood and social work practice have some relevance still today in terms of informing debates about the nature, quality and expectations of social workers' relationships with young children. These debates regarding the 'corporate parent' (that is, the nature of the professional caring roles and responsibilities for children in state care) are contentious (Leeson 2009). While there is not the room to summarize them here, nonetheless it is important to consider the broad issues as indicated through the exercise below.

EXERCISE

Consider the following questions:

- Are Sir Monckton's expectations regarding the social worker role realistic or too idealistic? Explore with examples from your own experience.
- What might be the impacts on social workers of implementing the model above?
- What might be the impacts on birth parents/main carers of implementing the model above?

Report of the Care of Children Committee: The Curtis Report (Curtis 1946)

The importance of a personal relationship between a social worker and children on their caseload was reiterated in the Curtis report that examined the care arrangements for children who lived in various types of residential facility. The care of children outside their family was of great concern in the 1940s in the UK. During the Second World War, the government organized the evacuation of huge numbers of children away from areas that were being bombed. Parents died during the war and many others had to abandon their children. Babies were adopted but most children lived in institutions. The Curtis Report (1946) investigated the conditions within a number of different types of institution including workhouses, public assistance children's homes and homes run by voluntary organizations, to name a few. In a summary of their general impressions about how some of the children were then cared for in some of the homes they specifically commented on the relationships between staff and children, noting that they were often characterized by a

> lack of personal interest and affection for the children which we found shocking. The child in these homes was not recognised as an individual with his own rights and possessions, his own life to live and his own contribution to offer. [. . .] He was without the feeling that there was anyone to whom he could turn who was vitally interested in his welfare or who cared for him as a person.
>
> (Curtis 1946: 134, para. 418)

Furthermore, in relation to children boarded out (placed with foster carers) they said that

> [t]here is no doubt that the O'Neill case had put authorities on their guard [. . .] and we thought that the individuals in charge were doing their best, though sometimes in a remote and impersonal way, to serve the interests of the children. But the present

administrative system seems to us full of pitfalls. Divided responsibility, office delays, misunderstandings and misjudgments of people, irregular visiting and failure to visit promptly in emergency, may easily under present conditions facilitate a tragedy, as they have done in the past.

(Curtis 1946: 135, para. 421)

In light of their investigations the Curtis Committee made 62 recommendations in its report, and on the 'personal relation' stated:

We attach great importance to establishing and maintaining a continuing personal relation between the child deprived of a home and the official of the local authority responsible for looking after him. [They should] be the friend of those particular children through their childhood and adolescence up to the age of sixteen or eighteen as the case might be.

(Curtis 1946: 147, para. 445)

The reports by Sir Monckton and the Curtis Committee therefore provide the very earliest evidence of a long-standing concern regarding failures in social worker–child relationships, some of the reasons why and how these led, in turn, to failures to protect, provide for and/or to encourage the participation of children. The implementation of the Children Act 1948 attempted specifically to address some of these problems through the creation of children's departments and children's officers. Children's officers were to meet the needs of children in their local authorities within the context of meaningful social worker–child relationships. The success of children's officers and the services that they shaped are exemplified through the working lives of women such as Barbara Kahan, Joan Cooper and Lucy Faithfull. For example, an obituary of Barbara Kahan stated:

She shouldered a caseload of her own, as well as managerial responsibilities. Nor was she past taking a child home for the night when no other place could be found. She was certainly an innovator. In Dudley, she opened the local authority's first children's home. In Oxfordshire, corporal punishment in homes was abolished in 1951, and imaginative fostering was introduced – 40 years ago, special rates were paid as an incentive for people to take difficult children.

(Philpot 2000: 1)

However, the introduction of the Local Authority Social Services Act 1970, with its emphasis on generic services and the generic social worker, brought with it the demise of children's officers.

Inquiry report into the death of Maria Colwell
(DHSS 1974)

Shortly after the reorganization referred to above, in 1973, Maria Colwell, aged 7 years, died following sustained neglect and physical abuse at the hands of her mother and stepfather, Mr and Mrs Kepple. While it appears that there was no direct connection between legislative changes and the death of Maria Colwell, events served to highlight ongoing concerns regarding the social worker–child relationship. During her first five months of her life, Maria lived with her mother. Mr and Mrs Cooper (extended family on the paternal side) then cared for her. Apart from one brief period when Maria's mother removed Maria from their care (threatened by the developing relationship between Maria and Mr and Mrs Cooper) Maria remained in the care of the Coopers until she was phased back home, aged 7 years, to the care of her mother and her new husband, Mr Kepple, in June 1972. Six months later Maria died having suffered chronic neglect and abuse in their care. On the evening of her death Mr Kepple had returned to the family home at 11.30 p.m. having spent the evening out. He found Maria downstairs watching the television. He kicked and beat her to death. In addition to pre-existing injuries, Mr Kepple's attack on Maria caused extensive bruising to her body and eyes, brain damage and other internal injuries to bones and soft organs. The pathologist described her injuries as 'the worst he had ever seen'.

A central concern to emerge in the subsequent inquiry (chaired by Mr Field-Fisher QC), which took place in 1973, was the lack of personal relationship between the social worker and Maria. Examples included: lack of visits by the social worker to Maria following her return home, failure by the social worker to engage with Maria and/or to see her alone when visits did take place, and an over-focus by the social worker on the parents rather than Maria.

The lack of a high-quality and personal relationship between Maria and her social worker permeated all aspects of the social service plans made for Maria. First, in the rehabilitation plan the social worker misunderstood and misinterpreted Maria's deep anxiety and unhappiness. As her visits to her mother and Mr Kepple became more regular, it was noted that

> Maria's resistance was becoming more strenuous, resulting in major scenes on nearly every occasion. Two visits had to be cancelled because she had worked herself into such a state of kicking and screaming that Miss Lees [social worker] realised it was impossible to insist.
>
> (DHSS 1974: 25, para. 54)

The social worker, however, did not actively explore or discuss Maria's feelings with her, refer her to someone more specialized or stop the rehabilitation plan. Instead she made a series of assumptions and guesses as to the cause of Maria's stress, which underestimated the distress and allowed the plan to proceed. On this the inquiry panel stated:

> We cannot accept that in a case such as this a child should be subjected to the degree of stress shown by Maria. Nor do we consider an intelligent guess as to the cause of that stress to be sufficient in this case [and that the social worker] had a right, indeed a duty, to consider and interpret Maria's feelings at this time [and that this is] a basic tool of her trade.
>
> (DHSS 1974: 27, para. 59, and 111, para. 318)

Second, the social worker was untruthful with Maria regarding the actual day when the return home was to take place. The inquiry report states that Maria went to school with her carer Mrs Cooper for the last time. This was unbeknown to Maria. Mr Cooper later collected her from school and took her to social services. It goes on to say that Maria had screamed and clung to Mr. Cooper at the office and was apprehensive about going with her mother who was present. She was given a reassurance by Mrs. Kepple in [the social worker's] presence that she would be returning to the Coopers at the weekend.

(DHSS 1974: 28, para. 64)

This was a lie with which the social worker actively colluded because the plan was that Maria would be returning home that day for good. Maria went home, never to return to the Coopers and in fact never to see them again. The inquiry panel stated, 'We think this was inexcusable' (DHSS 1974: 28, para. 64).

Third, following her return home in June 1972, Maria was not visited again by her social worker until December 1972. And yet during this time the concerns of neighbours and schoolteachers had grown. Fourth, when the social worker did visit Maria to investigate an injury, she was unsure 'as to whether she discussed the injury with Maria, that is heard any explanation from her own lips' (DHSS 1974: 41, para. 98).

In their conclusions and recommendations the inquiry panel devoted a section of their report to 'communicating with children'. They stated that

[o]ne aspect of Maria's story which has naturally given rise to concern is the extent to which the social workers directly involved in the case [. . .] were able to communicate effectively with Maria about her feelings, both during the period of transition and after her return home. It seems to us that this is a vitally important matter for all social workers responsible for children in care [and that] direct personal communication between social workers and children about their problems is indispensable.

(DHSS 1974: 76, para. 209)

The Colwell Inquiry demonstrated how weaknesses in the social worker–child relationship permeated all aspects of the social work process through from investigation, assessment and planning to decision-making and reviewing. Following the death of Maria Colwell, new legislation was introduced that increased the powers of local authorities in respect of children in their care. Known as the Children Act 1975, it was significant to the social worker–child relationship because it amended legislation regarding the separate legal representation of children in care proceedings in court. For the first time, it gave children in care the right to be consulted about decisions being made about them. The Children Act 1975 stated:

In reaching any decision relating to a child in their care, a local authority shall give first consideration to the need to safeguard and promote the welfare of the child throughout his childhood; and shall so far as practicable ascertain the wishes and feelings of the child regarding the decision and give due consideration to them, having regard to his age and understanding.

(Children Act 1975: section 59)

These legislative changes focused attention on the importance of the social worker–child relationship. Subsequent research by Page and Clark (1977), which drew attention to the dissatisfactions of young people in care about inadequacies of their relationships with their social workers, gave added weight to the demand for change in this area.

Further inquiries that took place between 1973 and 1981 (DHSS 1982) produced similarly depressing findings about the quality of social worker relationships with young children and a concerted desire to improve this. This desire was exemplified in an important social work text by Crompton (1980), which emphasized the social worker–child relationship. Crompton analysed reasons for the relative neglect of the relationship in social work training and practice and outlined practical steps that could be undertaken to improve practice to ensure that 'social workers should regard working directly with children as of prime importance' (Crompton 1980: 45).

Inquiry report into the death of Jasmine Beckford (London Borough of Brent 1985)

Despite these developments, ongoing failings in the quality of the social worker–child relationship were a feature in subsequent child abuse inquiries in the 1980s concerning Tyra Henry (died aged 21 months), Heidi Koseda (died aged 3 years), Kimberley Carlisle (died aged 4 years) and Doreen Mason (died aged 16 months). The most vivid of these, in terms of drawing attention to deficits in the social worker–child relationship, was the inquiry, set up and chaired by Louis Blom-Cooper QC, into the circumstances surrounding the death of Jasmine Beckford, who died when she was aged 4 years.

Up until she was 18 months old, Jasmine lived with her mother (Ms Beverley Lorrington) and stepfather (Mr Morris Beckford). In August 1981, at 18 months old she was admitted to hospital with a broken femur, which was deemed to be non-accidental. Her sister, Louise, also suffered non-accidental injuries at this time. Both were placed with foster carers and made the subject of care orders. In April 1982, Jasmine and Louise were rehabilitated home, still under care orders. By November 1982, the children's names were removed from the child protection register but the care order, which required social services to supervise and monitor the children, remained in force.

During that time Jasmine suffered a broken leg that went unnoticed by all of those involved in her care. In 1983, contact between Jasmine and the education and social services dwindled as she stopped attending nursery and was 'not present' when professionals visited the home. Jasmine was last seen alive by her social worker on 12 March 1984. At the post-mortem, Jasmine was noted to have suffered chronic neglect and abuse while living at home. It was later discovered that she had been locked in a room with bodybuilding weights tied to her legs to stop her moving. She had multiple injuries including burns, cuts and ulcers. Her ribs were also broken.

The catalogue of horrific injuries and incidents was testament, in part, to the failings in the social worker–child relationship. These failings became a central consideration in the subsequent inquiry in both the majority report (written by Field-Fisher QC and Davey for London Borough of Brent 1985) and the minority report (written by Stevenson as a submission as part of the main 1985 report, London Borough of Brent 1985). This inquiry resulted in the publication of two reports because there was a divergence of opinion in terms of explaining the failings in social work practice. The majority report focused more on the individual social workers involved while Stevenson, as she later explained (Stevenson 1986), although concurring with the overall findings, took a different perspective on explaining the failings. She drew attention to the social, economical, political and theoretical context of social worker decision-making. Stevenson's contribution was crucial in terms of opening up the debate about social work practice by urging people to look at the bigger picture.

In the majority report, the social worker's relationship with Jasmine was the subject of particularly heavy criticism because of a range of failings, including: infrequent visits, failure to engage and/or communicate with Jasmine on the few occasions when she was seen, focusing primarily on the parents rather than Jasmine and her siblings, and a failure to act decisively and use their authority vested in law to address these concerns.

With regard to the social worker–child relationship the inquiry panel stated:

> We wish to stress that the visits are to the children, and not to the parents [. . .] Ms. Wahlstrom [social worker] very seldom visited the Beckford family unannounced [. . .] We have, moreover, found that on no occasion over two and a quarter years of the home on trial did Ms. Wahlstrom take Jasmine out on her own for a walk; that she recorded no conversation with Jasmine; and that virtually all the entries in her Social Worker's Report which mentioned Jasmine were related to matters that occurred in the presence of one or both of the Beckford parents. Ms. Wahlstrom demonstrated with eloquent testimony the negation of any sense of the personal relationship between her and the two children.
>
> (London Borough of Brent 1985: 125)

The social worker's records bore witness to the lack of relationship with Jasmine. Here the inquiry panel stated:

> What is particularly lacking from both Ms. Wahlstrom's and Miss Leong's [health visitors] notes – particularly once the children had been returned home in April 1982 – is a record of either, or both of them, having exclusively focused their attention on the children, in particular on Jasmine. There is not a single entry that either worker ever spoke to the child, either alone or in the presence of her parents; there is no entry that either was looking for, or saw any sign of, possible further abuse. There is no entry that Ms. Wahlstrom ever took Jasmine out for a walk or saw her at school, other than on the one occasion in April 1983 when Beverley Lorrington was present.
>
> (London Borough of Brent 1985: 225)

The panel of inquiry made a forceful case regarding the failings of the social worker relationship with Jasmine when they concluded:

> Throughout the three years of social work with the Beckfords Ms. Wahlstrom totally misconceived her role as the field social worker enforcing Care Orders in respect of two very young children at risk. Her gaze focused on [the parents]; she averted her eyes to the children to be aware of them only as and when they were with their parents, hardly ever to observe their development, and never to communicate with Jasmine on her own. The two children were regarded as mere appendages to their parents who were treated as the clients.
>
> (London Borough of Brent 1985: 293)

Significantly they also took the opportunity to reflect beyond Jasmine's case and went on to state:

We fear that their attitude in regarding the parents of children in care as the clients, rather than the children in their own right, may be widespread among social workers. [. . .] It is axiomatic that the protection of the child can usually be best achieved by working with the family, of which the child is an integral part. But the *focus* must invariably be on the child. [. . .] Jasmine's fate illustrates all too clearly the disastrous consequences of the misguided attitude of the social workers having treated [the parents] as the clients first and foremost.

(London Borough of Brent 1985: 294)

The inquiry report highlights concerns in several interrelated areas of social work practice, including: social workers' lack of confidence in the legislative basis to their responsibilities; confusion regarding roles and tasks; poor inter-agency relationships; and the influence of the 'Rule of Optimism' (Dingwall *et al.* 1983). This refers to the tendency of social workers to reduce or minimize risk by being overly positive in their assessments of risks and parental capacity to change and assumptions about 'Natural Love' (the idea that parents love their children no matter what and would be the last to cause them harm).

In all this the social worker–child relationship was central because this was the site at which all these other factors coalesced. Stevenson, who produced the minority report into Beckford, accepted this, pointing out in later work that in a series of failings '[p]erhaps the most crucial issue of all [. . .] is the failure of the social worker to observe, assess and communicate effectively with children' (Stevenson 1986: 506–7).

Report of the inquiry into child abuse in Cleveland (Butler-Sloss 1988)

Concern over the rights of children to protection, provision and participation was also reflected in the Cleveland Inquiry chaired by Lady Butler-Sloss (Butler-Sloss 1988). The inquiry concerned 121 children living at home either with birth parents or foster-parents where a diagnosis of sexual abuse was made using controversial and contested physical medical evidence (reflex relaxation anal dilatation) (Butler-Sloss 1988). The inquiry findings revealed that social workers and others had over-relied on this evidence in deciding to remove children from their homes. By the time of the inquiry, 98 of the 121 children had been returned home. The inquiry made a series of recommendations about social work practice and cases of suspected sexual abuse, focusing on improvements in inter-agency cooperation, improved training and the early implementation of proposed new childcare legislation. Among the many recommendations made to the many involved professionals (including police and the courts), Butler-Sloss made specific recommendations regarding the social worker–child relationship in cases of sexual abuse. This was because she was concerned that during the assessment, planning and decision-making processes children had been overlooked. She stated:

There is a danger that in looking to the welfare of the children believed to be the victims of sexual abuse the children themselves maybe overlooked. The child is a person and not an object of concern.

(Butler-Sloss 1988: 12)

In this context Butler-Sloss stressed the rights of children to receive information appropriate to them about what was happening and why, be listened to, have what they say taken seriously, have their views to be represented in decision-making, and be protected from unnecessary intervention such as interviews and medical examinations. She also recommended that social workers should have full information about the children with whom they were working. Moreover, they should not make promises to children they cannot keep and they should ensure that at all times they acted in the best interests of the child(ren) concerned (Butler-Sloss 1988: 245). This inquiry report was again significant in highlighting how failures in the social worker–child relationship led to children being let down in terms of their rights to protection, provision and participation.

Research in the 1980s, regarding the implementation of the Children Act 1975 and of the mechanisms for statutory review of individual plans for children in care, also highlighted that few children attended their reviews (DHSS 1982; Adcock *et al.* 1983; CLC 1984; Sinclair 1984; Packman *et al.* 1986; Vernon and Fruin 1986). The research noted that there was limited evidence as to whether and how children had been consulted, and few observable mechanisms by which the views and opinions of children in care were included in decision-making processes. The effect on some children and young people in care was to leave them feeling disengaged, powerless and undervalued (CLC 1984).

The maxim from the Cleveland Inquiry 1988 – that 'the child is a subject and not an object of concern' – was reiterated in the Children Act 1989, which covered England and Wales. It was also reflected in the counterpart childcare legislation that was introduced in Scotland and Northern Ireland in 1995. The introduction of this childcare legislation was designed to bring about changes in the relationship between the state, parents and children. Importantly it centralized the children as individual subjects, persons in their own right as well as a members of their family and community. It sought to safeguard children and secure their well-being by ensuring that their rights to protection from harm, to provision of services/support and their rights to participation were clearly defined and legally enforceable. Through this new framework the social worker–child relationship was reconstructed to be closer to the role of the parent – responsible, accountable and central in terms of helping young children to secure positive long-term outcomes.

Report into the abuse of children in children's homes in Wales (Waterhouse *et al.* 2000)

However, further child deaths and subsequent inquiries in the 1990s continued to draw attention to the part played by poor social worker–child relationships in terms of securing the safety and well-being of children in their family homes as well as children in care (Levy and Kahan 1991; Utting 1991, 1997; Waterhouse *et al.* 2000). The Waterhouse Inquiry, for example, which focused on the abuse of children in residential homes in two former North Wales county council areas, stated of the social worker–child relationship:

> There was also a blatant lack of close personal relationships between residents and their field social workers [. . .] the overwhelming majority of residents complained of lack of contact with, and inability to confide in, their assigned social worker.
> (Waterhouse *et al.* 2000: 158, para. 11.52)

The lack of positive relationships made already vulnerable children much more vulnerable. The inquiry, in its concluding paragraphs, stated:

[I]t is necessary to stress here the importance of the duty of field social workers to establish and maintain a close relationship with children in residential care and to listen to their worries and complaints [. . .] Once a child is admitted into care, the field social worker carries the main responsibility for planning the future [. . .] In this context the development of a close and confiding relationship between social worker and child is of paramount importance and this, in turn, can only be established by regular visiting of both children in residential care and boarded out children.

(Waterhouse *et al.* 2000: 438, para. 29.60, and 446–62, para. 31.16)

Inquiry report into the death of Victoria Climbié (Laming 2003)

By 2000, there were many policy initiatives underway including the Quality Protects programme (DH 1998a, 1998b, 1998c; 1999a, 1999b), Learning to Listen (CYPU 2001) and the government's responses to this (DH 2002; Kirby *et al.* 2003) which were designed to improve the quality of care for children across a range of issues including their relationships with professionals and their involvement in decision-making. However, ongoing difficulties in day-to-day practice were again highlighted following the death of Victoria Climbié and the subsequent inquiry.

Victoria was born in Abobo, Ivory Coast, Africa. Victoria's great aunt, Marie-Thérèse Kouao, began caring for her in 1998. This arrangement was made with the consent of Victoria's parents, who believed that she would be well cared for and receive a good education. In about November 1998 the pair moved to Paris, France. It seems that Victoria was neglected and physically abused by her great aunt after their arrival in France. Victoria came to the attention of professionals because she was absent from school and then had her hair shaved and was wearing a wig.

In April 1999 the pair moved to London, England. They were in contact with social services for housing and financial purposes. Victoria was noted to look thin and poorly dressed in comparison with her great aunt but concerns were not high enough for social workers to take action. In July 1999, Ms Kouao met Carl Manning and he immediately moved in with the pair. In the same month Victoria was admitted to two different hospitals with non-accidental injuries. The misdiagnosis of these combined with the lack of discussion (by medical and social work staff) with Victoria about how the injuries had actually happened resulted in Victoria being discharged back to the care of Ms Kouao.

By August 1999, a social worker had been subsequently allocated Victoria's case. Although known to a social worker and other professionals Victoria died on 25 February 2000 of hypothermia in the context of malnourishment, a damp environment and restricted movement following the care she had received by Ms Kouao and Mr Manning. It emerged later that Victoria had spent days tied up by the hands and feet in a bin bag in the freezing-cold bathroom of the apartment she was living in. She endured beatings with shoes, coat hangers, hammers and bicycle chains. Neil Garnham QC (counsel to the inquiry), told the inquiry that when Victoria was fed,

[t]he food would be cold and would be given to her on a piece of plastic while she was tied up in the bath. She would eat it like a dog, pushing her face to the plate. Except, of course that a dog is not usually tied up in a plastic bag full of its

excrement. To say that Kouao and Manning treated Victoria like a dog would be wholly unfair; she was treated worse than a dog.

(Laming 2003: 1, para. 1.1)

The report of the inquiry into the death of Victoria Climbié was published on 28 January 2003 (Laming 2003). As summarized by Ferguson (2005), it highlighted a series of organizational failings that contributed to her death including: restricted resources and high caseloads; lack of training; poor inter-agency communication, cooperation and collaboration; poor supervision and training arrangements; and poor relationships within the social work team.

The report also highlighted that these organizational failings contributed to individual failings in the social worker–child relationship. Social workers' failings included: lack of visits to Victoria; failure to engage and communicate with Victoria in an individual and personal capacity when visits were made; and a failure to think through, articulate and act upon emerging concerns. The inquiry produced a report giving several vivid examples of the contribution of organizational failings to the failings in the social worker–child relationship. For example, when Victoria was in hospital in July 1999 a hospital social worker was allocated her case and was to undertake an initial assessment to clarify the nature of a possible child protection referral. The inquiry noted that

> Ms. Johns [the social worker] visited Rainbow ward on five different occasions but made no attempt to speak to Victoria. She [and other witnesses] gave several reasons why [they] did not. Several witnesses said they had seen guidance that said that they must be cautious about contaminating evidence or forming any kind of relationship with a child.
>
> (Laming 2003: 237–8, para. 8.97)

In relation to her practice, the inquiry stated that '[f]or any experienced social worker to believe that undertaking an initial assessment [. . .] could be done without seeing and speaking to the child [. . .] is difficult to credit' (Laming 2003: 237, para. 8.90).

After Victoria was discharged from hospital in August 1999 there were very few social work visits – four in total between August and her death in February 2000 (Laming 2003: 31, para. 3.49) with the total contact time being less than 30 minutes. When these visits did happen they were characterized by the social worker's lack of interest in or engagement with Victoria. The inquiry noted, for example, that on the second pre-announced social work visit 'Victoria seems to have been all but ignored [. . .] as she sat on the floor playing with a doll' (Laming 2003: 33, para. 3.59). The visits were also characterized by the social worker spending too 'much time [. . .] deferring to the needs of Kouao and Manning, and not enough time was spent on protecting a vulnerable and defenceless child' (Laming 2003: 205, para. 6.602). Furthermore, when the family became uncontactable in December 1999 and January 2000 the inquiry described the actions of the social worker as 'half-hearted' (Laming 2003: 189, para. 6.501).

The Laming Inquiry (Laming 2003) therefore drew attention to the fact that, in a context of broader organizational failings and at a crucial stage in Victoria's life, social workers had generally failed to see her alone, speak with her, listen to her or to seek her views. In the concluding sections of the report, Laming considers the position of the social worker relationship with the child. He states:

> There was general agreement that improvements are necessary in the way that staff

in the different services talk to children and how staff use the information given. A range of suggestions was made. However, a point that was returned to time and time again was the need for a relationship of trust between practitioner and child.

(Laming 2003: 353, para. 17.30)

Developments since the Laming Inquiry (2003)

Since the first Laming report (Laming 2003) there have been many significant legal, policy and practice developments designed to address organizational failings and to strengthen and improve the social worker–child relationship. These are, in part, based on the acknowledgement that similarities in the findings of inquiries over time are disturbing and that the situation has to change (Parton 2004). The Green Paper *Every Child Matters* (referred to hitherto as ECM) (HM Treasury 2003) provided the policy blueprint for more effective services for all children and their families. Following extensive consultation the government published *Every Child Matters: Next Steps* (DfES 2004b) and then passed the Children Act 2004, the legal framework by which the ECM: Change for Children programme would be implemented across all agencies and in respect of all children.

Under ECM and the associated Children Act 2004, the emphasis is on the integrated design and delivery of services based on commonly shared frameworks and tools for the planning, management and delivery of services to all children and their families. The success of services for children is measured against five outcomes, which all children should achieve. These are: being healthy, staying safe, enjoying and achieving, making a positive contribution, and achieving economic well-being.

Relationship is at the heart of children achieving these outcomes and the language of relationship underpins the recently introduced statutory guidelines (*Working Together to Safeguard Children* DCSF 2010b) for children at risk of harm, abuse and/or in need of support. For example, in the statutory guidelines it is stated that 'all agencies and professionals should prioritize direct communication and positive and respectful relationships with children, ensuring the child's wishes and feelings underpin assessments and any safeguarding activities' (DCSF 2010b: 32, para. 1.14). It also acknowledges that

> [s]ome of the worst failures of the system have occurred when professionals have lost sight of the child and concentrated instead on their relationship with the adults [and that therefore] the child should be spoken and listened to, and their wishes and feelings ascertained, taken into account (having regard to their age and understanding) and recorded when making decisions about the provision of services.
>
> (DCSF 2010b: 133–4, para. 5.5)

They further reiterate this by stating that 'children need to feel loved and valued, and be supported by a network of reliable and affectionate relationships. They need to feel they are respected and understood as individual people and to have their wishes and feelings consistently taken into account' (DCSF 2010a).

The non-statutory Common Core guidelines (DfES 2005), which have been designed by the Children's Workforce Development Council (sponsored by the DfES and other government bodies), and the National Children's Bureau training pack (NCB 2006) are relevant to all professionals working with children. They also emphasize the importance of professionals establishing trusting, consistent and long-term relationships, and state that 'continuity in relationships promotes engagement and the improvement of lives' (DfES 2005: 6). These have just been updated (CWDC 2010) again placing similar emphasis on the importance of the social worker relationship with children.

In relation to certain groups of children – specifically children in care – the *Care Matters* agenda is underpinned by an emphasis on the importance of relationship (DfES 2006, 2007; DCSF 2008a; DHSSPSNI 2008). At the time of writing, *Care Matters* is the most recent government policy initiative of relevance to all four UK jurisdictions providing a framework for all professionals who work with children in care to secure better outcomes for them by providing corporate (state) parenting based on high aspirations, stable relationships and listening to the voice of the child (DCSF 2008a).

This policy initiative has occurred during ongoing concern about the failure of children in care to achieve similar outcomes to their peers who are not in care. In explaining these failures, the focus has been on the failings of the state (in its role as the corporate parent) to carry out its parenting roles and responsibilities (the parent–child relationship) properly. Furthermore, children in care speak consistently about their lack of relationship with their social workers and the impact of this on them. In the Care Matters Consultation Response Document (DfES 2007), children and young people still feel that they do not have good-quality relationships with their social workers and that they are not listened to or included in their care planning. Children expressed concerns about 'not seeing their social worker enough, social workers not keeping appointments, social workers not having the power to make decisions and the huge turnover of social workers' (DfES 2007: 12). They also wanted their social workers to 'be effective, easier to get hold of, and [. . .] keep the promises they make' (DfES 2007: 13). The results of this latest document reflect other similar consultation exercises (ANV 2007; WMTD 2007).

In view of these concerns the *Care Matters* policy agenda, now enacted through the Children and Young Persons Act 2008, constructs the social worker–child relationship on a model of a positive parent–child relationship, very similar to that referred to by Sir Monckton in his report in 1945, and emphasizes that 'our aspirations for children in care are no less than those each parent has for their own children' (DCSF 2008a: 1). *Care Matters* urges that 'each organization should consider the quality of relationships it offers children in care and explore where improvements can be made'. It goes on to state that 'we will not be successful in improving outcomes for children in care' without attention to the importance of relationships. Social workers need manageable caseloads to allow them 'to invest time in building relationships with children' (DCSF 2008a: 13).

Several pilot initiatives are underway, under the auspices of the Children and Young Persons Act 2008 that are based on restructuring existing services and practices and aim to place relationships at the centre of social work practice with children. Initiatives include the Remodelling Social Work pilots, Social Work Practice pilots, social pedagogical approaches to the delivery of day-to-day care in children's residential homes and the rolling out of the Blueprint Project (VCC/NCB 2004) that aims to deliver a child-centred approach to planning and decision-making for children in care. The Children's Workforce Development Council, for example, is running the Remodelling Social Work pilot schemes. Eleven local authorities are involved in the pilot programme, which involves the reorganization of teams so that social workers can spend more time with children.

Social Work Practice pilots (being piloted by the government) are similar in that they involve a restructuring of social work teams along the lines of general practitioner practices, the aim being that social workers would be freer to spend time with children (Le

Grand 2007; DCSF 2008b; Winter 2009). In another development the government is funding a pilot study regarding the social pedagogical approach to the delivery of care in residential homes for children (with developments being reported on the supporting website, www.socialpedagogyuk.com). The child-centred approach is also the theme underpinning the Blueprint Project, whose roll-out, on a pilot basis, is being supported by Voice for the Child in Care and the National Children's Bureau (Voice 2010).

A further development is that, at the time of writing, the Children Act 1989 guidance has just been revised. The *Care Matters* White Paper set out some of the topics that now feature strongly in the new guidance. These include improving the relationship between social workers and children by ensuring that children are usually seen alone without carers present and putting arrangements in place for children to contact social workers outside scheduled visits (DCSF 2010b). Many of the developments are also encapsulated in the Children and Young Persons Act 2008.

Finally, in relation to practice, many materials and resources have been made available to enable social workers to better communicate with children. Most notably, these include National Children's Bureau *Listening for Life* leaflets, the Blueprint Project and Participation Works, which defines itself as the 'online gateway designed to improve the way practitioners, organisations, policy makers and young people access and share information about involving children and young people in decision making' (taken on 5 May 2010 from www.dcsf.gov.uk/everychildmatters/strategy/participation/participation/).

Report into the death of Peter Connelly ('Baby P') (Haringey LSCB 2009)

Despite the renewed emphasis on the importance of the social worker–child relationship, the profession was recently rocked once more by the death of a child known to social services, in this case Peter Connelly (Haringey LSCB 2009) who was born on 1 March 2006 and died on 3 August 2007. Peter was also known as 'Baby P', in attempts to keep his identity confidential during court proceedings. He died at home, aged 17 months, having suffered chronic neglect and physical abuse at the hands of his mother and stepfather. He had suffered over 50 injuries by the time of his death and a post-mortem revealed that he had a broken back and ribs, that the tips of some of his fingers were missing, nails missing and that he had swallowed a tooth having been punched. Throughout his short life numerous professionals including social workers and health visitors had visited him. One of the simple and yet understated facts of the case is that it appears that not one professional had a good enough, close enough relationship with Peter to 'connect' with him, to assimilate the signs of abuse and to act decisively on them. The Laming report that followed the death of Peter has said of the social worker–child relationship:

> It is important that the social worker relationship, in particular, is not misunderstood as being a relationship for the benefit of the parents or for the relationship itself, rather than a focused intervention to protect the child and their welfare.
>
> (Laming 2009: 23)

Lastly the most recent biennial review of serious case reviews (Brandon *et al.* 2009: 40) reinforces the centrality of the social worker relationship when it speaks of the 'invisible

child'. The report states that, '[f]rom within the spectrum of inter-connecting fɐ
one overarching theme dominates the enduring problem of the child being "lost
the theme of children not being seen or heard is a feature of most studies of serous cɑɔᴗ
reviews' (Brandon *et al.* 2009: 40).

The government response (DCSF 2009a) to the Laming report (2009) states:

> Crucially, Lord Laming has stressed the importance of placing the child at the centre
> of all that we do. That means understanding the perspective of the child, listening
> to the child and never losing sight of the child. Just as the centrality of the child
> drives our policies so too should it drive day-to-day practice at the front line.
>
> (DCSF 2009a: 4, para. 6)

It is these sentiments that underpin the new statutory guidance for all professionals
working together to safeguard children (DCSF 2010b). In a section of the guidelines
entitled 'The Child in Focus' there are a series of actions that professionals should
undertake to put this sentiment into action. These include (among others): developing a
direct relationship with the child; obtaining information from the child about his or her
situation and needs; eliciting the child's wishes and feelings – about their situation now
as well as plans and hopes for the future; providing children with honest and accurate
information about the current situation, as seen by professionals, and future possible
actions and interventions; involving the child in key decision-making; and providing
appropriate information to the child about his or her right to protection and assistance
(DCSF 2010b: 33–4, para. 1.18). The following chapters in this book address directly
each of these main action points and provide practical examples of how social work
practice with young children could be transformed.

Summary

The analysis of official inquiries and serious case reviews has shown that remarkably
similar concerns have repeatedly been raised for over 50 years regarding the quality
and nature of social worker relationships with young children. These concerns, located
within the context of broader organizational failings, constitute significant shortcomings
in social work practice. These include failures by social workers to: visit the children
frequently; to engage and communicate with the children or to see them alone when
visits did take place; to think through and articulate verbally or in records their concerns; to act decisively upon visible cumulative concerns especially children's weight
loss, neglect, bruises and behavioural disturbance; and above all to make the child the
focus of the intervention instead of focusing on the parents.

This litany of failings can feel overwhelming, hard to digest and difficult to translate
into practice. However, it is important to remember that the worst failings relate to a
very small number of cases. Having said this, it is also important to think about the state
of social work practice more generally and to ask the question, 'do children known to
social services get the best from their relationships with social workers?' In asking this
question I am mindful that publicity about the inquiries described above has tended to
focus more on individual social worker failings and less on the organizational issues
that constrain social work practice with young children. The fact that the nature of
the failings have remained so consistent means that there are broader organizational
factors – associated with the nature and role of social work – that also need to be taken

into account and these will be explored in Chapter Three. This is not to discount the influence of individual attitude and ideology as most social workers would say that they would like to be able to do more to build relationships and communicate with young children and that they are aware of the value of those relationships. This is the theme of the next chapter.

2 The importance and value of relationships

Summary of chapter content

This chapter explores why relationships between social workers and young children are so important. It also considers what qualities, inherent in those relationships, are valued by both social workers and children and concludes by drawing attention to the major sources of frustration as identified by social workers and young children building and maintaining good relationships.

Introduction

As was seen in the previous chapter, there have been long-standing concerns about the state of social workers' relationships with young children. This chapter looks in more detail at why social worker relationships with young children are so important and also what young children value in those relationships. Before doing this, however, it is important to begin with an outline of what is understood by the term 'young children' and what is known of the characteristics of the young children that come to the attention of social services. This is essential if we are to understand why social worker relationships with them are so valuable and important.

Young children known to social services

Often when social workers talk about young children it is assumed that everyone knows what is meant by the term 'young children'. However, social workers will have come across several definitions depending on which professionals they are talking to. For example, if social workers are liaising with workers in pre-school settings those professionals will be referring to young children as pre-school children, typically aged 3–4 years, whereas in primary school settings teachers will either be referring to young children as those between the ages of 4 and 11 years or specifically those who are in Key Stage 1 (KS1) (i.e. 5- to 8-year-olds). For the purposes of clarity, this book uses the definition outlined in a UN report that states that young children are

> all young children: at birth and throughout infancy, during the pre-school years; as well as during the transition to school. Accordingly the Committee proposes the period below the age of eight years as an appropriate working definition of early childhood.
>
> (UN: 2005, para. 4)

Children of these ages become known to social services for a variety of reasons including: being at risk of harm, in need of support, involved in court proceedings and/or in care. Some of these young children are called 'looked-after' children, which is a legal term in the UK that refers to those placed in care on a voluntary basis or a legal order and subject to statutory review processes, whereas others are not. Some young children are living at home with their parents/main carers and others are living with extended family, foster carers or in residential care. In addition, some children's names are on the child protection register (confidential list of names held by social services of children who are believed to be at risk of significant harm) and others are not. Recently published statistics on children 'looked after' in England (DCSF 2009b) indicate that children under 9 years of age make up nearly a third of the total looked-after child population.

The main reason that children come to the attention of social services is because of abuse and neglect. Other identified reasons include family dysfunction, absent parenting, acute stress in the family and/or illness/disability of parent or child. Over half of the total looked-after child population in England is the subject of a full care order (where the local authority or trust has acquired parental responsibility through the court process). Nearly three-quarters of all looked-after children in England live in foster placements with most of those foster placements being provided by the local authority (DCSF 2009b).

In terms of placements, while the figures indicate that 10 per cent of all children have experienced three or more placements it was also the case that 67 per cent of all children who had been 'looked after' for the previous two or more had stayed in the same placement. While the figures for Scotland (Scottish Government 2010), Wales (Welsh Assembly Government 2009) and Northern Ireland (DHSSPSNI 2010) are broadly similar there are some variations reflecting differences in legislation, policy and procedure. For example, in Scotland, by virtue of the different legal framework, the most recent figures indicate that 39 per cent of children 'looked after' were placed at home with parents and 20 per cent were cared for by friends or relatives (Scottish Government 2010). This is higher than elsewhere. Furthermore, figures in Northern Ireland draw attention to the fact that a lower proportion of the total looked-after child population is the subject of a full care order although this has been increasing year upon year (DHSSPSNI 2010).

Research indicates that before coming into care young children are particularly vulnerable given their family circumstances, their own needs and their care experiences. In terms of their family circumstances research indicates that young children often come from families where there has been a constellation of difficulties including: parental substance dependency; mental/physical ill health; domestic violence; as well as poverty, isolation, poor housing, unemployment and/or single parenthood (Bebbington and Miles 1989; Cleaver *et al.* 1999; Monteith and Cousins 2003; Winter and Connolly 2005; Ward *et al.* 2006). In the course of their young lives, and before coming to the attention of social services, they may have already experienced several changes in carer (Ward *et al.* 2006; Ward 2009).

On entry into care young children are more likely to experience emotional and behavioural difficulties (Monteith and Cousins 2003; Sempik *et al.* 2008) including bedwetting, aggressive and challenging behaviour and sexualized behaviour. Furthermore, they are more likely than children in the general population to experience health and education difficulties. For example, in relation to health, Monteith and Cousins (2003) noted that, of their sample, 56 per cent had health problems including asthma, developmental

delay and visual/hearing impairments. Once in care some young children struggle edu-
cationally (Greig *et al.* 2008) and their difficulties can be compounded by experiences
such as placement instability (Ward *et al.* 2006) and delays in decision-making about
permanent placements in the court system (Ward *et al.* 2006: McSherry *et al.* 2006;
Munro and Ward 2008; Masson *et al.* 2008).

The particular circumstances and experiences of young children outlined above highlight that young children known to social services are therefore highly likely to have
experienced some abusive, chaotic, fractured, frightening and violent relationships.
As Sempik *et al.* (2008) and Schofield (2005) have highlighted, these experiences have
already impacted on children's emotional and behavioural development by the time
they actually enter the care system. Seen in this context children's relationships with
their social workers are crucial in terms of helping children begin to address, make
sense of and successfully move on from these issues.

The importance of the social worker relationship

Social workers should already have a good understanding of the value, desirability
and importance of meaningful relationships with young children. For example, in their
training, social workers are introduced to a range of theoretical approaches that draw
attention to the importance of positive relationships in a child's life. These theoretical
approaches, drawing from a range of disciplines including developmental psychology,
social psychology and sociology, include concepts such as attachment, resilience and
socialization. Together they capture the necessity of a child having: secure attachments
with significant others (including parents/main carers); the importance of a child having
the opportunity to learn and model out the behaviours and social norms of positive
role models around them (including immediate family, friends and those in educational
and social settings); and the significance of a child having the opportunity to exercise
choice and contribute to their relationships with others (including friends, peers and
so forth).

Unfortunately, there is no space within this book to explore in-depth these theoretical
approaches but for those interested good introductory guides are provided by Trevithick
(2005), Aldgate *et al.* (2006) and Horwath (2009). However, it is still important to note
how these frameworks have tended to inform and define social worker practice and,
in particular, how they have encouraged social workers to focus primarily on the need
to develop, maintain and enhance the quality and stability of *other people's* positive
relationships with young children (be they carers, relatives, friends, teachers, peers and
coaches) and to protect children from harmful and abusive relationships. In so doing
it has often been the case that the quality and significance of the social worker's *own
relationship* with the child in question has received less attention and less priority either
in social work training or in subsequent practice. This fact, as seen in Chapter One,
has been noted in many of the reviews of social work that have taken place following
the deaths of children known to social services, including those of Victoria Climbié
and Peter Connelly, and has led to the development of a series of pilot projects aimed
at enhancing the significance of the social worker–child relationship. A further related
development is the renewed emphasis on relationship-based social work practice in
social work literature notably, and most recently, by Ruch *et al.* (2010) that explores
the broader theoretical concepts and processes associated with relationship-based social
work practice more generally.

EXERCISE

Think about your own relationships with others in general and consider the following:

- How big is your own relationship network?
- What positive relationships, if any, did you have as a child? Why are these important?
- Did you have any negative relationships as a child? If so, what do you feel have been some of the adverse consequences of these?

So why is the social worker relationship so important? To address this relationships will now be considered in terms of their contribution to: long-term positive outcomes for children; effective implementation of social work processes; and securing the protection, provision and participation rights of young children. Crucially, the perspectives of the children who are known to social services will also be considered with regard to these issues.

Positive relationships and children's long-term outcomes

The idea that children are more likely to achieve positive outcomes if they have stable, positive and long-term relationships with those around them is at the heart of the *Care Matters* agenda which, at the time of writing, is being rolled out in England, Scotland and Wales (DfES 2006, 2007; DCSF 2008a; DHSSPSNI 2007) and, in England, has been enacted through legislation in the Children and Young Persons Act 2008. Positive outcomes for young children include attention to their health, education, employment and social and emotional well-being. While the *Care Matters* agenda refers specifically to children in care it has broader implications for social workers and their relationships with young children who are known to, but not necessarily in the care of, social services.

The government urges all those professionals who work with children to fully understand their responsibilities towards children. The type of relationship it argues should be aspired to is that of 'a good parent who looks out for [children], speaks on their behalf and responds to their needs' (DCSF 2008a: 7, para. 1.3). The relationship should be characterized by three core components: 'high aspirations; stability; and listening to the voice of the child' (DCSF 2008a: 7, para. 1.2). As noted in the exercise in Chapter One, while there are questions as to whether this type of relationship that is modelled on the social worker being, in effect, the child's parent is appropriate, realistic and/or achievable, the government is designing frameworks and services based on this model.

It is with this in mind that government policy makes clear that it is the responsibility of all professionals, including social workers, to work towards better outcomes for children by appreciating the value of their own relationship with the child and by working in ways that reflect this. While the policy agenda makes reference to the importance of field social workers (those in teams in offices) where it notes that they 'need to have manageable case loads that allow them to invest time in building relationships with children' (DCSF 2008a: 13, para. 1.16), it singles out the importance of children's relationships with residential social workers, stating:

Where these attachments are good we know that children are happier and have better outcomes [. . .] The best carers understand children, rewarding good behaviours and modelling more appropriate approaches where necessary. The quality of care provided has a crucial effect not just on stability of relationships but also on health, well-being and education.

(DCSF 2008a: 11, para. 1.12)

This view is supported by other research with children in care that states:

There is a body of research about children [. . .] which demonstrates the positive effects of good relationships on a child's development. High self esteem, resilience and positive outcomes are associated with a child having at least one high quality relationship with an adult in their lives.

(VCC/NCB 2004: 37)

Writers indicate that, for children in care, particular areas of their emotional and social well-being that require special attention and that rely on stable and positive relationships include children's identity, sense of belonging, completeness and continuity of their life story (Schofield 2005; Winter and Cohen 2005; Luckock *et al.* 2008). Social workers cross the paths of children at difficult points in their lives. Their relationships with children have particular significance for that reason. They often act as a bridge providing continuity between the past and the present for the child. The importance of this cannot be underestimated. In building up their life stories children require information about the events, places and people of their histories. In terms of this identity construction young children often listen to other people's 'stories' and memories ('I remember when you were two and you . . .') and then use them to construct their own story of their past ('when I was two I . . .').

For some children it is the field (team-based) social worker who can help in this process having been a part of the child's life historically. Sometimes it is not the foster carers or the residential social workers who have had access to the child's past but it is a social worker. Even though there is a high turnover of social workers it is still they, with access to full historical records, who have the potential to help children clarify and confirm their views and experiences of their past. The social worker should be in a position where, through their continuous relationship, they can bring insight and understanding in response to the child's questions and anxieties about the past (Why did that happen? Who was there? What did they do? What did they think? Did they love me? Who am I?). This may help children build a stronger sense of their own identity, provide them with a sense of belonging and contribute to their emotional well-being (Winter and Cohen 2005; Luckock *et al.* 2008).

It is within this context that, as noted in Chapter One, the government is investing significant funding in pilot projects that are restructuring the design of services to emphasize the importance of high-quality social worker relationships with children. It is the government's view that this will help children achieve more positive outcomes in terms of their health, education and social/emotional well-being. Despite the fact that evidence is still required, through evaluations of these projects, to substantiate this view it is important to highlight these precisely because they are influencing and informing policy and service design.

Positive relationships and effective social work processes

Social workers will be familiar with social work processes which are defined as: investigating and assessing, planning, decision-making and implementing, reviewing and evaluating (Watson and West 2006). The effectiveness with which these processes, whether in relation to children at risk, children in need or children in care, are carried out by social workers relies on building meaningful relationships and communicating effectively with children. Moreover, all the related statutory guidance highlights that social workers must complete investigations and assessments that are a valid, accurate, clear and inclusive reflection of children's circumstances (CWDC 2009: 23). They also highlight that to achieve this social workers need to develop meaningful and good-quality relationships with the children concerned.

Table 2.1 provides a summary of the different groups of young children that come to the attention of social services, the social work processes that will be instigated in relation to them, the statutory guidelines that govern those processes and the references to the importance of the social worker relationship contained within those guidelines. It is worth briefly looking at each of these groups of children in turn.

Children at risk

As is shown, social work intervention regarding 'children at risk' (child protection) cases is governed by statutory guidelines. In England and Wales these are the most recent *Working Together to Safeguard* guidelines (DCSF 2010b), which state clearly that, in the management of individual cases,

> [t]he child should be seen (alone when appropriate) by the lead social worker in addition to all other professionals who have a responsibility for the child's welfare.

Table 2.1 Statutory guidelines and social worker relationships

Children	Social work process	Statutory guidelines	Relationship
Children at risk	Investigation and assessment	*Working Together to Safeguard Children* (DCSF 2010b)	A relationship based on seeing the child, keeping them in focus and hearing their voice (DCSF 2010b: 132).
Children in need	Investigation and assessment	*Framework for the Assessment of Children in Need and their Families* (DH *et al.* 2000)	A relationship based on direct work and of seeing, observing, talking, doing and engaging with the child (DH *et al.* 2000: 43).
	Assessment and planning	*Common Assessment Framework* (DfES 2004a; CWDC 2009)	A relationship based on full involvement of the child in formulating solutions and decision-making (CWDC 2009: 19).
Children in care	Planning, decision-making, implementing, reviewing and evaluating	Statutory guidance for children in care (DCSF 2010c)	A relationship based on engagement with the child to develop their strengths and resilience (DCSF 2010c: 9–10).

His or her welfare should be kept sharply in focus in all work with the child and family. The significance of seeing and observing the child cannot be overstated.

(DCSF 2010b: 82–3, para. 5.5)

Similar guidance is available through the devolved administrations of Scotland and Northern Ireland (DHSSPSNI 2003; Scottish Executive 2004a, 2004b). The English and Welsh guidance goes on to state that children's consent should be sought and that decisions made about them should be made with their agreement, bearing in mind their age and their level of understanding, unless to do so would place the child at risk of significant harm. Furthermore, as noted in Chapter One, the guidance (DCSF 2010b) provides a breakdown of all the ways that professionals can keep a child in focus including: developing meaningful relationships with children; respecting their rights to information, participation and protection; and communicating with children to gain their wishes and feelings. The following chapters show, in practical ways, how this can be achieved in day-to-day social work practice with young children.

Children in need

In relation to children in need, the *Assessment Framework for Children and their Families in Need* (DH *et al.* 2000) clearly states that

> [d]irect work with children is an essential part of assessment as well as recognizing their rights to be involved and consulted about matters which affect their lives [. . .] There are five critical components in direct work with children: seeing; observing; talking; doing; and engaging.
>
> (DH *et al.* 2000: 43)

The more recent Common Assessment Framework (CAF) (DfES 2004a) is a shared standardized framework for use by all professionals working with these children. Its purpose is to promote the early identification of children with additional needs (as opposed to being at risk of harm) and the coordination of integrated services to meet those needs. Its aim is preventative in that it seeks to help children 'before things reach crisis point' (CWDC 2009: 11) and/or to 'stop children slipping through the net' (CWDC 2009: 15). In completing an assessment it is emphasized that

> [t]he CAF is entirely voluntary. You must discuss your concerns with the child or young person and/or their parent/carer before deciding on a common assessment. The child or young person and their parent/carer, where appropriate, are key to effective solutions so must be involved in their design.
>
> (CWDC 2009: 19)

Furthermore, the informed and explicit consent of the child or young person and/or that of their parent/carer must be secured before completing an assessment, before sharing information with other professionals and before securing provision from identified services (CWDC 2009: 20). A similar version of the Common Assessment Framework known as Understanding the Needs of Children in Northern Ireland (UNOCINI) is available in Northern Ireland (DHSSPSNI 2008). In Scotland another similar framework, known as Getting it Right for Every Child (GIRFEC), has also been recently implemented

(Scottish Government 2008). In the guidance accompanying the UNOCINI there is a very strong emphasis on the centrality of the social worker–child relationship:

> To maintain a child-focused approach, the child must be seen and kept in focus throughout the assessment. Account must always be taken of the child's perspective and this attention must not be diverted by the many other factors that may be encountered when working with families. Speaking with the child, or using another form of communication, to assess their needs and circumstances is central to gaining an understanding of the child [. . .] The significance of involving the child in the assessment process cannot be overstated. An assessment should tell the child's story and provide an overview of their wishes and feelings, their hopes and fears. In the majority of circumstances, it will be essential to share assessment and planning information with the child. It is not acceptable to take decisions to withhold information purely on the basis of age or understanding [. . .] attempts must be made to include the child and work in partnership with them at all times.
>
> (DHSSPSNI 2008: 9)

Children in care

With regard to children in care, the review and care-planning processes and the powers and duties of local authorities in England, Wales and Scotland (and trusts in Northern Ireland) are set out in childcare legislation: The Children (Northern Ireland) Order 1995; Children (Scotland) Act 1995; and in England and Wales the Children Act 1989 as amended by the Children (Leaving Care) Act 2000, the Adoption and Children Act 2002 and the Children and Young Persons Act 2008, and the accompanying regulations and guidance. In England, new care-planning, placement and case review regulations came into force in 2010. An e-consultation document produced by the government outlines the importance of the social worker–child relationship when it states:

> It is particularly important for children to feel that they are active participants and engaged in the process when adults are trying to solve problems and make decisions about them. When plans are being made for the child's future, they are likely to feel less fearful if they understand what is happening [. . .] There are further practical reasons for ascertaining children's wishes and feelings: many children have an understanding of what is causing their problems and what underlies their needs; they may have insight into what might or might not work in the context of their current circumstances and environment; they often know what sort of support they would most value and be able to access; engaging children helps to recognise their difficulties and develop their strengths and to help promote their resilience.
>
> (DCSF 2009b: 9–10)

What the guidelines do, in relation to all the various groups of children, is to stress the importance of social workers engaging in relationships with children where they involve children meaningfully and ensure that their perspectives are central to all parts of the process. Weak social worker relationships clearly have a detrimental impact on these processes and also, as discussed below and later in the book, constitute a failure to respect, uphold and honour the indivisible and interdependent protection, provision and participation rights of children that are outlined in the United Nations Convention on the Rights of the Child (UNCRC) (UN 1989).

The importance of relationships in securing children's rights

The United Nations Convention on the Rights of the Child – hitherto known as the UNCRC (UN 1989) – defines children's rights to provision, protection and participation. The UNCRC is an international convention that the British government is a signatory to, along with nearly all other countries in the world, and that both defines the rights of children and creates obligations on 'state parties' (i.e. governments and government organizations and agencies) to ensure that those rights are respected, protected, promoted and fulfilled. Within this, children are known as 'rights holders' and governments are known as 'duty bearers' (O'Neill 2008: 10). Parents, who are specifically mentioned in the UNCRC, are both duty bearers and rights holders. Social workers, in acting on behalf of a legally and governmentally sanctioned statutory organization, have a responsibility to understand children's rights, to be clear about what rights are being breached and, like parents, to develop with children ways of ensuring that they can exercise their rights in line with their evolving capacities.

Within the UNCRC provision rights refer to children's rights to services, support and information. Particular provision rights include those for health needs (article 24), social security (article 26), standard of living (article 27), education needs (articles 28, 29), rehabilitative care (article 39), those in juvenile justice systems (article 40), as well as provision of guidance, information and support (articles 13, 17, 42).

Rights to protection refer to protection from harm, abuse and exploitation and include protection from kidnapping (article 11), all forms of violence, abuse and neglect (article 19), from drug use and/or involvement in production and distribution (article 33), from sexual exploitation (article 34), from sale, trafficking and abduction (article 35), from exploitation (article 36), from torture and deprivation of liberty (article 37) and from war and armed conflict (article 38). Specific groups of children requiring special protection include those children without a family (article 20), being adopted (article 21), who are refugees (article 22), with disabilities (article 23), and/or those children involved in child labour/work that threatens their education, health and development (article 32).

Rights to participation include children's right to receive and impart information, in a media of their choice, to express their views, to have their views taken into account, to be represented in decisions about their own lives and to enjoy freedom of thought, conscience and religion (articles 5, 12–17). Although separated out for the ease of description it is important to note that children's rights are indivisible and interdependent. This means that they cannot be viewed and implemented in isolation from each other.

Positive meaningful relationships between children and adults are essential in enabling children to secure their rights, especially their participation rights. Indeed, article 5 of the UNCRC places parents and state parties under a duty to support children in doing this. The importance of the UNCRC in developing social worker relationships with children will be explored further in Chapter Four.

Children's views about relationships with social workers

EXERCISE

Before reading on in this chapter, consider the following questions:

- What views do you think children express about their relationships with their social workers?
- What positive qualities do you think children experience?
- What frustrations do you think children have regarding their relationships with social workers?
- Do you think children are realistic in terms of what they want in their relationships with social workers?

While it is clear that the importance of social worker relationships with young children is now formally recognized by government and reflected in its priorities and policies, and that the principles underpinning meaningful relationships are enshrined in the UNCRC (UN 1989), it is clear from research with children that there remains a long way to go in terms of these principles being reflected in day-to-day social work practice. In this final section, the findings of a considerable body of research that has sought children's perspectives about their relationships with their social workers will be considered. What this shows is that children want meaningful relationships with their social workers (DfES 2007; CWDC 2009). The Children's Workforce Development Council, responsible for improving the standards and practice of all those working with children, has recently stated that '[c]hildren and young people [. . .] expect their social worker to establish and maintain stable and respectful relationships, to listen to them and promote their interests' (CWDC 2009: 1).

Some children have been able to establish meaningful relationships with their social workers, which were very important to them (Buchanan *et al.* 1993; Fletcher 1993; Lynes and Goddard 1995; Thomas and O'Kane 1998; Munro 2001; Bell 2002; VCC/ NCB 2004; NICCY 2006; Morgan 2006; Leeson 2007; McLeod 2006, 2007, 2008a, 2008b). For these children they tend to value relationships with their social workers because these mean that someone genuinely takes an interest in them, wants the best for them, enjoys being with them and is also concerned for them (McLeod 2008a, 2008b). This is confirmed, for example, from findings of a study that focused on children's perspectives about being in care where it was reported that '[a]ll the children mentioned the importance of the social worker in their lives. The social worker was seen as very powerful and, when the relationship worked well, as a very strong ally' (Munro 2001: 131).

In other research regarding the perspectives of children in care about their experiences, it was noted that children appreciated certain qualities in social workers including them being 'funny', 'friendly', 'nice', 'considerate' and 'a good person' (Fletcher 1993: 16) as well as having a 'genuine interest [. . .] meeting up [. . .] as arranged, getting things done as agreed, being open and honest, and maintaining links with young people's families' (Baldry and Kemmis 1998: 133). The views of children on the importance of their social worker are encapsulated in a research review summary by Hill (1997: 56) that focused on the perspectives of children in care:

The studies in this review demonstrated how important were both the *interpersonal role* and *personal qualities* of social workers. Young people said 'they had been influenced by the advice and guidance of their social workers to modify their offending or addictive behaviour but *only after a relationship of trust had been built up*. We also found that for some young adults seeking to manage alone after leaving care, the social worker was a life-line, giving both practical help and moral support.

Not surprisingly, the research also highlights the frustrations, disappointments and negative experiences of children in care and their relationships with their social workers (McLeod 2001, 2007; VCC/NCB 2004; DfES 2007; Leeson 2007; Morgan 2006; ANV 2007; WMTD 2007). A combination of problems has significantly marred the processes of forming and maintaining relationships for some children. These include: inconsistency (erratic, infrequent timing of visits), instability (changes of social worker) and unreliability (social workers failing to turn up to appointments or failing to carry out agreed tasks because of workload demands). These are problems that social workers are all too aware of. In more recent research carried out by the Blueprint team – a team within the voluntary organization Voice for the Child in Care (VCC) that sought the perspectives of children in care and professionals looking after them – one social worker said:

> The worst thing about this job is that you don't get enough time to spend with children. The time is taken up with filling in forms, paperwork and meetings about things that sometimes seem a long way from a direct service to children.
>
> (VCC/NCB 2004: 2)

Instability of relationships is not helped by the organizational practice in social work of moving cases between teams. As noted in the same research,

> [g]ood relationships with professionals are squandered. Children and young people want to be able to maintain relationships with staff that have worked well. From a staff point of view the main reason for cutting off contact is not their use of time, but a view that maintaining relationships is unprofessional and lacks boundaries. We are working in a culture where emotional distance is seen as an essential part of a professional approach.
>
> (VCC/NCB 2004: 47)

The report goes on to state:

> Every child who is looked after should have a person who remains in contact with them throughout the period they are in care and beyond. This person (named the BFG [Big Friendly Giant] by one young person) should be chosen by the child and could ideally come from their existing network. If there is no obvious candidate then the child would be helped to find someone, possibly someone who has worked with them in a professional capacity, or someone who is specially appointed to be their BFG.
>
> (NCB/VCC 2004: 47)

The impact on children of these difficulties in their relationships with social workers is also well documented. As a young person in a report by Morgan (2006: 28) has argued,

> [i]t's not rocket science! Kids just want to be wanted because when you are in care you feel like no one wants you. You just want people to listen, understand and be there on a regular basis so you know that you've always got something to hang on to. It's not too much to ask!

These frustrations are shared by other children who are not in care but who are known to social services, who need support and/or are at risk of harm. When their views have been sought it is apparent that, at times, the lack of any meaningful relationship has negatively impacted on the assessment, planning and decision-making processes for them (Holland 2004; Cleaver *et al.* 2008). Cleaver *et al.* (2004: 95) state that, from their interviews with children,

> few understood the process of assessment, or could remember whether a social worker had explained to them what would happen and why. They reported difficulty talking about personal issues with social workers and felt that what they said was frequently discounted and disbelieved.

Summary

This chapter has illustrated that the quality of social workers' relationships with young children has been a concern for some time. Relationships are now a central theme in government priorities and policies and are seen as crucial in terms of encouraging children's well-being and development, respecting their rights and ensuring effective social work practice. There have been useful policy developments, in the form of statutory guidance, that also place value on these relationships. However, it is known from official inquiries and also from the perspectives of the children themselves and their social workers that social worker relationships with young children continue to cause concern. Why do all these failings persist? It is crucial that social workers have a rounded and full view of the factors that act as barriers to them building relationships and communicating with young children and this is the focus for the next chapter.

3 Barriers to building relationships

Summary of chapter content

It is argued in this chapter that the set of taken-for-granted assumptions and practices that social workers tend to operate by – that can be called their professional habitus – is crucial to understanding the barriers that exist in relation to them building meaningful relationships with young children. This chapter identifies and outlines seven key barriers – tasks, trust, threats, theories, training, tools and time. Pockets of good practice, which draw attention to atypical practice are used to argue that barriers can only be effectively challenged by a combination of changes at both the individual and organizational levels.

Introduction

> Throughout our inquiry, one theme emerged as particularly dominant: the importance for children in care of stable, reliable, nurturing relationships with those who care for them and manage their care. The failure of the care system to replicate or compensate for the stable relationships that most children have with their parents is one of its most serious and long-standing deficiencies. Even when all the right frameworks and structures are in place, it is the quality of relationships that will determine whether a child in care feels cared about on a day-to-day basis.
>
> (HC CSF 2009: 27)

One thing that stands out from the overview of the findings of the many different inquiries outlined in Chapter One is that, regardless of the time period or the particular events described, the nature of social workers' relationships with young children and their day-to-day practices have remained remarkably consistent. This is so even though the inquiries span many decades and focus on social workers operating in a range of different places. The purpose of this chapter is to look at why this is the case. What will be seen is that social workers tend to share a number of taken-for-granted day-to-day practices that, in turn, can be seen as reflective of the broader organizational and structural norms of the social work profession.

Traditionally two types of factors have been identified in attempts to unravel the causes of poor social worker–child relationships: organizational factors (such as the high caseloads that social workers carry and, therefore, the lack of time they can spend with an individual) and individual factors (the characteristics of particular social workers, such as their lack of confidence, skill and/or knowledge). Unfortunately, the relationship between these organizational and individual factors, and, more specifically, exactly how one informs the other, has not been fully explored and developed in the research literature. However, unless we can develop a better understanding of the relationship between an individual social worker's practices and the structural factors that come to inform and shape these then it is likely that there will be no significant changes in social workers' relationships with young children.

It is with this in mind that the chapter begins by looking at the broader organizational contexts within which social workers operate and how these contexts, over time, come to inform and shape social work practice. In particular, it will be shown how social workers progressively come to adopt a set of often taken-for-granted ways of thinking and behaving in response to the broader structures and pressures they are under. It will be suggested that the disposition to respond to situations in particular ways can be regarded as a set of unconscious habits that, because they tend to be common to many social workers' practice, can be termed their 'professional habitus', to borrow and adapt a concept from the French sociologist Pierre Bourdieu (see Bourdieu 1972). Having outlined the broader organizational structures within which social workers operate, the chapter then focuses in more detail on the nature of their professional habitus itself and the particular taken-for-granted ways in which social workers tend to think and behave in their day-to-day work. By drawing upon in-depth interviews with social workers that were conducted as part of the broader research study outlined in the introduction to this book, the chapter will show that there are a series of barriers that tend to undermine social workers' relationships with young children.

EXERCISE
Before moving on, consider briefly the following questions:

- What do you think are some of the main barriers facing social workers in being able to develop meaningful relationships with children?
- Think about how you would attempt to address some of the barriers if you were a social worker, a social work team manager and/or a policy maker.

Barriers to developing meaningful relationships

In considering social work practice there are many potential barriers to establishing meaningful relationships with young children. For the purposes of clarification in this chapter I have identified various barriers and have labelled them as the 'seven T's' (adapted from Winter 2009) that comprise: tasks, trust, threats, theories, training, tools and time (see Figure 3.1).

It is important to note that these barriers are not being held up as typical, in their entirety, of all social work practice. Nor do they appear uniformly in all social work practice. Rather, the purpose of the chapter is to identify and explain some of the most commonly occurring barriers that are likely to be present to differing extents and in different combinations among individual social workers. The chapter will now consider each barrier in turn and explain its nature and influence on the professional habitus of social workers.

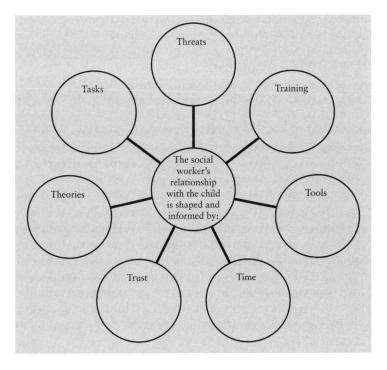

Figure 3.1 Factors affecting relationships between social workers and children.

Tasks

The nature, purpose and functioning of the social work profession has recently undergone an extensive set of reviews (Asquith *et al.* 2005; Bogues 2008; GSCC *et al.* 2008; Blewitt *et al.* 2007; DCSF 2009c, 2009d). These reviews have drawn attention to the fact that there is a difference between the role of social work (i.e. its purpose) and the tasks of social work (i.e. the activities designed to achieve its purpose and its intended outcomes). At its most general level, the General Social Care Council (GSCC) has defined the purpose of social work as being to: secure and enhance the well-being of individuals and families, promote social change and enable people to reach their full potential (GSCC *et al.* 2008). To achieve this social workers are required to carry out several interrelated tasks including, among others, bureaucratic tasks, assessment tasks and social control tasks (Asquith *et al.* 2005: 2–3). The feeling among many social workers is that these tasks they have to perform reflect the growing emphasis on bureaucratization and managerialism (Ruch 2010a: 22–5) and tend to hinder their ability to develop effective relationships with young children (Le Grand 2007). These are each explored briefly below.

Bureaucratic tasks

There are three elements to bureaucratic tasks that form a barrier to social worker relationships with children. First is the lack of time available to social workers. The Social Work Task Force emphasized this when it stated:

> We have been told that social workers feel [. . .] tied up in bureaucracy. [. . .] They feel that they spend time on administrative tasks, which are not a good use of their skills and take time away from high quality casework.
>
> (DCSF 2009d: 1)

This concern is shared by others (Houston and Knox 2004; Asquith *et al.* 2005; Gupta and Blewitt 2007; Le Grand 2007). For example, Le Grand (2007) notes that

> social workers [. . .] come to work with a strong sense of moral purpose, idealism, energy, enthusiasm and commitment to rectifying injustice. However, once into the job, social workers often feel de-motivated, overwhelmed by bureaucracy and paperwork and deprived of autonomy.
>
> (Le Grand 2007: 17)

This lack of time can clearly have an impact on social work practice with young children. For example, and in relation to the present research, some social workers said that, because of bureaucratic tasks, they visited children less often and also communicated directly with children infrequently. They felt that they had to ensure that the statutory and procedural requirement to see the child (not necessarily talk with the child) had been met and recorded on the appropriate statutory form. For example, during her interview with me, Celia (a social worker) described the pressures as follows:

KW: So for you and other social workers what is the priority when you do home visits?

Celia: It is to actually see the children; so you can say that you have seen them. So that the statutory bit of the job is done; you know in your case file you can say: 'did visit, saw children, children OK'.

KW: [. . .] But there is no section dedicated to the views, story as told by the child?

Celia: No, no there isn't. You see the priority is to do your 'stat' home visits and there are loads of these. You haven't got time to spend individual time with each child.

Celia's comments reflect the increased bureaucratic emphasis that many social workers feel is placed on meeting targets and form-filling (DCSF 2009d; Ruch 2010a, 2010b). It has, therefore, become an acceptable practice, and one legitimated by recording requirements, that a social worker can visit a child, and record that they have seen the child, without actually having communicated with them in a meaningful way. To the extent that this has become a taken-for-granted practice common among social workers; it can also be seen as constituting part of their professional habitus.

In addition, this can also be seen in relation to the completion of consultation forms that have been designed for use by social workers to communicate directly with children to ascertain their wishes and feelings. However, because of the pressures of time and demands of workload, some social workers have adopted the practice of simply delegating their completion to foster carers, thus removing another opportunity provided for direct contact with the child. This is illustrated in the comments by Gillian, another social worker:

Gillian: Em, they [children in care] do get the consultation papers and they fill those in. They normally fill them in with their foster carers [. . .] but they are always aware that their meetings are going on and as I say they would, they have filled in their consultation paper, which has been good.

This statutory task should be undertaken by the social worker. It is also clear that its delegation to others reduces the opportunity for social workers to build meaningful relationships and communicate with young children and potentially discover vital details about carers and the quality of daily care. However, it is also not surprising that, in an organization where there are high caseloads and the emphasis is on targets and form-filling, this practice has developed and become a taken-for-granted aspect of many social workers' practices or a part of their professional habitus. The emphasis on form-filling is clear from the accounts of children themselves when given the space to describe their feelings about their social workers. For example, Leeson (2007) noted, following an interview with a young person in care, that

> social workers did not care about the children in their care, that they were more concerned with paperwork, fulfilling obligations that he was not aware of and being seen to do something.
>
> (Leeson 2007: 273)

Furthermore, other researchers in their interviews with social workers noted their concern that

> paperwork and inputting of data into management information systems were seen to now dominate the work of social workers [who] felt this left little time for building relationships with children and families, which was their primary motivation for entering the profession.
>
> (Gupta and Blewitt 2007: 174)

Assessment tasks

As noted in earlier chapters, assessment is a core task in social workers' practice (Holland 2004; Aldgate *et al.* 2006; Horwath 2009) designed to ascertain vital information about children and families where children are at risk of harm, in need of support and/or in care. It is therefore one of the main avenues through which a relationship between a child and a social worker is established. To this extent research has indicated that through the assessment process there has been an increase in the *quantity* of direct contact between children and their social workers (Holmes *et al.* 2009) and, since the introduction of the most recent assessment frameworks (in particular the Common Assessment Framework), an increased number of children appear to be involved in these assessment processes (Cleaver *et al.* 2008). However, the social workers participating in the present study identified that there are two barriers to forming relationships with young children in the task of assessment: anxiety about causing children harm/distress and anxiety about parents' reactions.

As regards the former, while social workers generally understood the organizational priority to complete assessments, the actual process of involving young children in completing assessments was hindered for some because of a concern about the potential emotional risk to children of talking with them about sensitive issues. Gillian, for example, explained her anxiety during her interview:

KW: Do you think it [involving children in assessment and decision-making proc-
           esses] could do any harm?
Gillian: I think that with regards to harm, my only concern is for the younger ones
           being there, involved. For example, I mean if it had, had to be discussed
           why mum didn't attend the family centre and the reasons for that [. . .] can
           those kids take on board why the mum didn't do that? Are those kids going
           to go home thinking 'mummy can do nothing for me'.
KW: So in terms of [involvement] it's partly about the information being shared
           and then the impact that it would have on the children?
Gillian: If there was a potential for it to be harmful then [it would be] emotionally.
           I'm thinking of Grace [a young child] you know [and if] the incidents were
           brought up [. . .] How would she have felt sitting there? You know [. . .]
           is she going to go home and dwell on this and with her age [is it] going to
           impact on her emotionally?

This anxiety about causing harm to young children by talking with them about personal issues is noted in other social work literature. For example, Schofield (2005) in her work has discussed the difficulties experienced by children who are known to social services and where exposure to neglect, abuse and violence has affected their ability to form relationships and to identify, explore and manage their own emotions and feelings. Given these issues there is a concern that involving young children in conversations to explore their feelings could reawaken hidden abusive memories and contribute to fresh behavioural and emotional disturbance if left unsupported. This concern is not confined to the social work profession. Alderson (2000/2008: 70) points out that 'people not in favour of consulting with young children tend to feel: deep concern about children's vulnerability; [and] anxiety that children are [. . .] a potential danger to themselves and others'.

   In the present research the other barrier identified by the social workers in forming relationships with children was the reactions of the parents. Inquiries have shown that where parents are suspicious or ambivalent they are more likely to view the social workers' attempts to talk with their children as a threat (Laming 2003). In these cir-cumstances some parents may also exert a lot of pressure on their children to say or not to say certain things in their meetings with social workers. Some social workers were worried for the safety and well-being of the children as a consequence, as Celia explained:

KW: Why do you think the parents won't let you talk with Crystal and Conor
         [children]?
Celia: Well I guess it's because they are afraid of what the children might say; you
         know they might spill the beans about what's really going on at home or
         something like that.
KW: So do you think that Crystal and Conor might have things to say?
Celia: Yes. They probably might if they were given a chance but that is the other
         worry. I don't think it's a good idea to take the children out and see them by
         themselves because of the way the parents react; you know I took Christine

[older sibling] out by herself last week and we had a great time. Or so I thought. It wasn't long after I dropped her back home that her parents were on the phone saying I had said this and that to Christine, which I hadn't said. They got the wrong end of the stick about everything; that's the difficulty working with these parents, as you know. They hear things and then totally twist them around; it's as if they are trying to twist the children's minds against anyone trying to get close to their children.

KW: Is that all the children?

Celia: Yes and if you think about it, it would be worse for the younger ones because there's more of a worry that they keep things less well hidden and that when they got home, if they ever saw me by myself, just imagine what pressure they would be put under to say what they had said to me. That's another reason for not seeing the younger ones by themselves; it just puts them under too much stress and pressure. It's good to know what children are thinking but you have to think about how their parents might think to what their children have said. You might put them at more risk.

As a result of these concerns, part of the social work professional habitus has been the practice of tending to avoid involving children where there is perceived resistance. A consequence of this is that social workers do not fully engage with children during social work assessments, planning and decision-making. Similar themes are noted elsewhere. For example, Holland (2004) considers the representation of children in assessments based on the framework Assessment of Families and Children in Need and found that 'children were [. . .] minor characters in the narrative' (Holland 2004: 73). Examples included describing children to 'fit with checklists, such as developmental milestones' (Holland 2004: 84) rather than fully engaging with the child as a person.

On the one hand the practice of avoiding engaging with young children because of these anxieties does seem to be 'common sense' because it might be seen to be in children's best interests, and allay the fears of their parents, to shield young children from talking about a complex array of emotions. However, on the other hand, this aspect of the professional habitus of social workers effectively serves to silence young children, and inhibit and detach social workers from relating and listening to them. The relative silence of children in assessments has more recently been highlighted through research into the processes and practices surrounding the use of the Common Assessment Framework (CAF) (Pithouse 2006; Gilligan and Manby 2008; Pithouse *et al.* 2009). For example, Gilligan and Manby (2008: 183) note that

[i]n contrast to government rhetoric emphasising the desirability and need for their involvement, for most of the children and young people, the process of CAF assessment was one in which adults talked about them rather than one in which they [children] were full participants.

Social control tasks

Finally, in terms of the tasks that social workers are required to perform, it is important to consider what happens to social workers' relationships with young children when they operate as agents of social control. Being an agent of social control refers to the legal mandate of the social worker job, which necessarily involves statutory intervention into the private world of the family. This intervention can, for example, result in the removal of children, the placing of children in alternative care and the imposition of restrictions around family contact. While carrying out these tasks, it can be very difficult for social workers to build relationships and communicate with young children, especially where the child disagrees with the intervention of the social worker or with the care plans or the restrictions. This was evident through the present research and, in particular, the lack of trust that some of the children felt towards their social workers which, in turn, discouraged them from wanting to develop relationships with their social workers. *Trust* is therefore another identified barrier for social workers. This can be seen below where social workers, first Haven and second Gillian, describe how they feel that children view them negatively when they have to keep children from their families.

KW: Or, does Heather [child] have a different coping mechanism maybe which is this, the shutdown?

Haven: Yeah.

KW: Kind of switch off?

Haven: The only person I would say she's really chatting to is her key worker who is doing a one-to-one with her which at least she has someone.

KW: Yeah.

Haven: To, but I find, as a social worker, a fieldwork social worker, those kind of one to one, you know, counsellor kind of environment, you don't really have because you're the person who is deemed to be the person keeping them from their families.

In a separate interview, Gillian further explains:

KW: Do you, do you think the children perceive of you as a trusting figure or?

Gillian: I think Grady [child] probably will always see me as the person that came and took him away from his mummy. I think that's his only, that is the only way he can understand that.

Another example of the difficulties for social workers in building relationships with young children when carrying out tasks associated with being an agent of social control is where social workers believe that children perceive them as always bringing 'bad' news as illustrated in the following interview excerpt with Haven:

KW: Has he ever said anything that he's wanted that you've been able to do for him?

Haven: [. . .] even the mobile phone, they're saying no to that [. . .] and that's why I think he is [like he is], 'cause I'm always the bearer of bad news, I'm always the one going out and putting the barriers.

KW: Putting the barriers down?

Haven: I couldn't blame the child for disliking you, you know.

Haven's thoughts are a reminder of how difficult it is to form a meaningful relationship with young children in care when they perceive that the social worker is always working against their wishes rather than for them. This is further highlighted below where Haven uses the example of moving one of her children, Henry, between placements against his will and the profound impact that had on their relationship. Henry, who did not want to move, lost all trust and hope in his relationship with Haven when he was moved against his will, as she explains:

KW: Do you think that's some of Henry's problem? That he feels that he's not being listened to?

Haven: God, he's had so many placements, a lot of them, like, he, he didn't want to leave Hammond Square residential unit, and he told me he didn't want to leave Hammond Square residential unit, and he was then off in tears, and I still had to move him and Henry resented me for that and I think Henry does think, he doesn't trust social workers.

Children's views about their social workers obviously inform their views about whether they wish to talk with them or not. There is a dilemma for social workers here because on the one hand the UNCRC underscores the need to respect a child's choice not to talk and yet, on the other hand, social workers do have a statutory duty to talk with young children. McLeod (2007) in her research with older children in care noted that some children displayed a range of negative behaviours in the interview process, which included anything from avoidance (not turning up at all) through to resistance and denial during interviews that did take place. McLeod concluded that these behaviours represented attempts by children to regain control over what they viewed as adult-imposed agendas and where their experience had previously been that social workers did not listen to them or offer them choices. She concludes by stressing the importance of social workers' relationships based on a deeper understanding of the inherent unequal power dynamic. At a practical level this would include building up trust over time and encouraging children to operate more control and choice in their meetings with social workers.

Related to this, McLeod (2007) makes a very important point about the need to reflect more on the reasons for children's non-engagement. What appears to happen sometimes is that children's negative responses are taken at face value by the social workers and used as the reason to invest no further in the relationship. In such circumstances, social workers' perceptions of children's views about them can therefore become part of their professional habitus, and can reinforce practices of less investment in building relationships because it is perceived that children are not receptive to these.

Threats (to self)

Alongside *tasks* and *trust*, a third barrier to social workers developing meaningful relationships with children are *threats* or, to be precise, threats to self. The practice of 'keeping one's distance' from young children seems to be further reinforced by social workers' perceptions of the 'risk to self' and their anxiety about ever-present threats of complaints, accusations of negligence, failure, loss of reputation and dismissal (Parton 2006; Green 2007). The emphasis on personal risk has increased anxiety and the development of a range of taken-for-granted defensive practices (Parton 2006; Ferguson 2005; Webb 2006; Green 2007; Ruch 2010a, 2010b).

In the present research the threat of violence from some families was also a significant barrier to building relationships and communicating with children. This is not a new finding, however. Stanley and Goddard (2002) interviewed workers from 50 child protection cases where children were living at home on orders and found that in the six months preceding the interview a significant number of workers reported serious incidents of actual or threatened violence, including: 23 who had experienced a death threat, 13 who had been physically assaulted and 43 who had been threatened in some way.

However, it is not just the level of violence that can act as a barrier for social workers but also how they manage their emotional responses when confronted with violence. In this sense, Stanley and Goddard (1997, 2002) apply 'hostage theory' to help understand why, where workers are faced with evidence of violence to children, they do not act. The hostage theory is also known as the 'Stockholm syndrome' and, as Stanley and Goddard (1997: 47) explain, 'describes where, under conditions of extreme threat, isolation and powerlessness the hostage or victim may unconsciously [. . .] engage in self-deception with the result that the relationship with the perpetrator may move from one of fear or anger to ambivalence and then perhaps to understanding'. With reference to social work practice, what this means is identification and cooperation with the abuser may increase the social worker's safety but also increases their feelings of powerlessness. The end result is a failure to challenge the abuser or to form an alliance with the victim (the child). To the extent that this response forms part of the taken-for-granted practices of social workers, then this aspect of the professional habitus will clearly act as a barrier to forming relationships with children.

Ferguson (2005) demonstrated the power of this aspect of the professional habitus by applying the model to the Victoria Climbié case, described in detail in Chapter One. He states that Victoria's carers (Ms Kouao and Mr Manning) 'dominated professionals [and that professionals then] behaved like their slaves – or "captors". Unconsciously, workers mirrored Victoria's feelings of terror and took up the "servant" position that they observed Victoria taking' (Ferguson 2005: 789). While on the one hand this response is understandable, Ferguson argues that the crucial issue for social workers is to be able to reflect on the feelings evoked by their contact with families because if they feel fear and terror it is likely that the child involved feels fear and terror too. However, it was found in the present research, as will be seen below, that social workers tend to be offered no or very little space and support to fully reflect on their emotional responses to families and children.

In the present research some of the social workers defined 'threats to self' as also including loss of reputation (as an objective, detached professional) if they expressed strong emotions in response to the intensely sad, challenging and difficult circumstances faced by young children. In the research some of the social workers wanted to protect themselves from becoming emotionally over-involved in and possibly overwhelmed by children's very unhappy circumstances. Some social workers managed these emotional and psychological risks to self by developing taken-for-granted routines which reduced the opportunities for exposure to emotional interactions with children, and therefore the likelihood they might display strong emotion.

One avoidance routine that constituted part of their professional habitus was to maintain distanced relationships with the young children based on a 'this-is-difficult-to-bear-and-therefore-best-not-to-hear' approach. Ferguson (2005) notes a similar response by professionals to Victoria Climbié. While professionals did know about some of Victoria's abuse as they saw the injuries, they did not necessarily act. It could be argued that their 'professional paralysis' may possibly be explained in part by their unprocessed emotional responses to Victoria and her circumstances.

In the present research it was found that the research interview was sometimes the only opportunity social workers had to explore and reflect on their emotional responses. During the interviews I noted that they experienced a number of emotions including: sadness, anger, compassion, empathy, hate, disgust, relief, hopelessness and shock about the young children's experiences but that they also lacked the space to address the impact of these emotional responses on their relationships with young children. In the example below, Lorraine discusses her emotions and coping mechanisms following the removal of three children from extremely neglectful parents.

Lorraine: When we finished the visit we sat in the car in complete silence. We just couldn't believe what we had seen. It was beyond belief that behind an ordinary looking front door you could walk in to such filth. It was stinking too. I mean stinking. I went home with the smell still in my nostrils [. . .]. It was like I had become contaminated or something. It didn't leave me. I couldn't eat or sleep. I felt sick you know heaving like [. . .] It gets worse when you hear snippets of what the children are saying cos it's like it was like a living hell for them [. . .] part of you wants to hear it because you can hardly believe it, curiosity like, but the other part says 'no don't go there it's too much, it's not normal' and then you block it off cos you have to, to cope with the next crisis.

Social workers' unwillingness to engage explicitly with the emotional aspects of their work, as seen in the example above, does reflect organizational professional norms of being detached, objective, balanced and unemotional. Practices reflective of these norms become part of their professional habitus and can then act as a barrier to building relationships and communicating with children (Leeson 2007, 2009). These barriers are then reinforced by related organizational practices, which include an increased reliance on the statutory completion of forms and where then supervision is dominated by ensuring that the statutory requirements have been met. This changed emphasis is described in this interview with Kirsty:

Kirsty: I think that people come into social work, they want to do that work with children and they want to spend time with them, but it just slips down [the] list of priorities.

KW: Do you think there are any [. . .] barriers?

Kirsty: I suppose if it was something [coming] through management as 'this is very important' whereas the way social workers are managed, it's more about meeting deadlines and 'Have you got this done? Have you got that, have you thought about that report?' There wouldn't be very much about your direct work with children and young people and how you feel about it.

Theories

The professional habitus of avoiding engaging in relationships with young children, as described above, is further reinforced, explained and justified by age-related assumptions about them. This leads us to the fourth 'T' – *theories* – or, in this case, theories of the incompetence of young children. In this respect it is interesting to note that recent government guidance promotes a view of young children as capable and competent:

With young children, the social worker should be creative and imaginative in finding ways to communicate with the child and discover his feelings. All children need to be given information and appropriate explanations so that they are in a position to develop views and make choices.

(DCSF 2010a: 5)

However, the present research revealed that social workers, in their day-to-day practice, did not always reflect this position. In fact, social workers' reliance on the completion of age-related child development pro formas (during assessment and review) created a tendency in practice, first to objectify children as a fixed set of records rather than attach value to subjective and relational child–social worker interactions and then, second, to underestimate the capacities and capabilities of young children by virtue of their age (as also noted in the work of Holland (2004)).

Some social workers felt that they did not need to spend much time investing in relationships with young children who were assumed to feel less, ask less, demand less and understand less than older children. Furthermore, younger children were perceived as not knowing what was going on, as unreliable, changeable and therefore untrustworthy. Briege highlights examples of these assumptions held by social workers about young children's incapacities in the following discussion:

KW: Is there the possibility that younger children are more able or advanced than people think they are or?

Briege: Possibly, but [. . .] the younger the child is, you think it's easier because you think, 'Well, emotionally it's not going to impact on the same'. I would rather remove a 4-year-old than remove a 9-year-old because I imagine their understanding and their loss is greater.

KW: Really?

Briege: Yes, probably, and I hate removing maybe 12-year-olds who are feeling rejected completely, you know, and it's really, I'd rather remove a 2-year-old, a 4-year-old.

KW: And do you, do you think that that perception is right that younger children experience less loss or less?

Briege: Maybe. God forgive me, you know what I mean, you know, it's really that you don't have to give an explanation 'cause they're not going to ask you, whereas the older child will ask you, you know, it's very, very difficult, and I think probably that is where, it is difficult, you know.

Some social workers also tended to undervalue and underestimate children's views by defining them as unreliable, based on misguided loyalty and unduly influenced by parents. In the next example Briege reflects on young children in care who state a desire to return home. She believes that children are not free to say that they want to stay in their placements but that it is more socially acceptable to say they wish to go home.

KW: You attend a range of meetings, so you will come across these forms. Do you find them useful?

Briege: I think it's very difficult for children to be put on that spot because are you getting a, you know, a truthful answer? Because most children will say to you, 'I want to go home' or they may not express their views about their placement just as honestly as they possibly could.

This issue was expanded upon in a separate interview with another social worker, Fiona, who could not understand why the child she was working with, Finn, wanted to return to the family chaos from which he had been removed. She queried the validity of his view by suggesting that he had an unthinking loyalty and was unduly influenced by his mother.

KW: The children [. . .] they're saying they want to go home?

Fiona: I suppose as a social worker, as a person, I don't know how a child would want to go back into that chaos.

KW: So it's difficult for us as outsiders to understand why you would want to do that?

Fiona: I think, I mean, your family are your family [. . .] you can't replace your mum [. . .] and they are who they are, but to what extent he wants to be involved again I'm not sure, and he has great potential now and he has settled well in Flamingo Place [. . .] I think there is that loyalty or there's just that almost 'push the button' automatic response and [. . .] there's a lot of influence from his mum.

The tendency of some social workers to underestimate the potential of young children to have understanding and insight into their circumstances can also be seen as an element of their professional habitus and creates a barrier to meaningful relationships and communication. There is also a tendency for some social workers to undervalue the potential contributions young children can make in explaining their experiences and their needs. To dismiss children's accounts justifies the taken-for-granted beliefs and practices as to why it is not necessary to invest heavily in listening to them and encouraging them to trust and to talk. The influence of age-related assumptions about children's poor level of understanding and insight are all pervasive themes, seen in this interview with Celia:

KW: With regards to Crystal [aged 5 years] and Conor [aged 8 years] was any information provided to them?

Celia: Not directly no. I don't think they really had any idea what was really going on.

KW: Were there any reasons for this?

Celia: Well it's mainly about their age. Crystal and Conor are too young to really understand what is going on. Um; I think they are not really competent. I mean don't have the insight.

These taken-for-granted assumptions about young children form part of the professional habitus that tend to be unstated, seldom acknowledged and therefore unquestioned and thus act as powerful organizing principles of practice (Holland 2004; Taylor 2004). They appear to significantly deter some social workers from attempting to form relationships with this group of children. This is despite the fact that there is a wealth of evidence demonstrating the capacity, competence, insight and understanding of younger children (Alderson 2000/2008). Even though some social workers may generally accept this view they, and others, identify the lack of training and tools as a further barrier to building relationships and communicating with young children.

Training

Some social workers highlighted that their relationships with young children were also hindered by a lack of availability of *training*, the fifth 'T' to be considered here. Unpublished research by the Children's Workforce Development Council Research Team (2009) on the perspectives of newly qualified social workers notes that 'many social workers believe their training fails to prepare them for working with families in crisis' (2009: 11). Following the death of Peter Connelly, the House of Commons Select Committee on the Training of Social Workers report opened by stating:

> When social workers are poorly trained – lacking in knowledge, skills or experience – or left unsupported in highly pressured situations, children's lives are put in danger.
>
> (HC CSF 2009: 3)

Lord Laming, in his report, said:

> The message of this report is clear: without the necessary specialist knowledge and skills social workers must not be allowed to practise in child protection.
>
> (Laming 2009: 4)

The training of social workers is currently a government priority in England in particular and incorporates several strands: previous qualifications and relevant practical experience prior to course entry, degree curriculum content, quality of practice placements; newly qualified social worker programmes and post-qualifying training. In all areas recommendations for change have been made by Laming (2009), the Social Work Task Force (DCSF 2009c, 2009d) and the House of Commons Children, Schools and Families Select Committee (HC CSF 2009) to ensure that

> as far as possible they [staff at the front line] put themselves in the place of the child or young person and consider first and foremost how the situation must feel for them.
>
> (Laming 2009: 22)

Recently published work (Luckock *et al.* 2007; Lefevre *et al.* 2008) indicates the view that there must be a concerted effort within social work training to prioritize communication skills with young children by developing a model that combines knowledge, skills and values and that is integrated into and embedded in all aspects of the degree programme.

Tools

The lack of available *tools* that social workers can use to communicate effectively with children represents the sixth barrier to be considered here. In relation to the present research, for example, social workers highlighted a dearth of materials, resources, dedicated physical space, facilities and a lack of creativity often relying on forms to structure their relationships and communication with young children. These issues, combined with a lack of training, had a negative impact on social workers' relationships with children as seen in this discussion with Briege:

KW: We've kind of discussed some of the limitations and problems with different methods, but do you think anything could be done differently?

Briege: I have to say, it's all about how the form and [how it] is structured, it's about the worker and their preparations for it [and there's] very little training in that.

KW: I was going to say, is there much training?

Briege: Very little, very little.

KW: Do you get to do any?

Briege: Not really, you know. Not specifically how to communicate with a child in care [. . .] how to respond to a child who is wanting more contact, that you can't give them, and how you create a situation where you can explain the reason why, but in a way that's going to be age-appropriate, [. . .] giving you examples of how you apply that to specific cases.

Moreover, in the following discussion, Kirsty highlights that it is not just training but also confidence to use the skills and knowledge acquired that affect the practices of some social workers:

Kirsty: I think that it's like everything, I suppose, you know, you need to develop your skills in communicating with children, and albeit that you get some interviews that are relatively straightforward and they go very smoothly and the child is the type of child who wants to open up and tells you lots of things, equally you can have children who are very closed, and that's going to be more intensive work and you need to be more creative [. . .] I'm just a wee bit afraid that I'll try something that doesn't work at all or that in some way causes the child more distress and anxiety and that's not what I'm trying to do.

Kirsty also highlights that social workers need opportunities to develop relationships, to build mutual confidence and to test out different or new ways of working with young children. The lack of time reinforces those practices, that have come to form part of the social work professional habitus, where building relationships and communicating with children remains underdeveloped and avoided.

Time

More generally, in the present research, a seventh 'T' that was highlighted as a barrier was *time*; it acted as a significant constraint on social workers' ability to build relationships with young children. Lack of time to build relationships with young children appears to be partly caused by the time-consuming nature of completing bureaucratic tasks (Gupta and Blewitt 2007; Bogues 2008), but also partly caused by wider resource constraints in which social workers are allocated very high caseloads, making it impossible to spend individual time with children and develop relationships with them (Laming 2003). Briege describes such pressures in this interview excerpt:

KW: One of the other problems you've highlighted is time?

Briege: You know, well, if you're going out to a family of four children in one placement and you have to do that [get the form completed] with all of them, it's very, very time-consuming, you know, children aren't getting home from school till half three, the social worker maybe has children [and has to be] out of the office at five so it's time-limited in terms of what you can do.

Gillian expands on this point in another interview:

KW: Are, and are there barriers to getting individual time [with] the children?
Gillian: I think from, from my point of view there are barriers because there are [so many] children in this family. Em, and I think it's a caseload, it's nearly a caseload in itself and to do it properly and to do it justice you, you need so much more time than you have.
KW: And they're not [placed] together?
Gillian: They're not together so you're flicking between one and the other. It's just very difficult. Em, if you had those children on their own with no other cases I mean you could get in there and get so much done. Em, but, but that hasn't been possible until now. And now the children are having to be referred to other agencies for their individual working you know but that, that sort of I feel, because I, I know them so well I suppose that that would've been my em, but that's just not possible you know.

To address the resulting gaps in their own relationships with children, social workers rely on other staff, such as key workers, residential social workers, foster-parents and counsellors. This can tend to lead to children experiencing fragmented relationships with a range of people, and no one taking an overall view, as highlighted by Fiona in the following discussion:

Fiona: The family are very new to us so I suppose it's about finding out what life has been like for those children, just in a general way but in saying that, I haven't been able to, and that, those are pieces of work I'd like to do, but at the minute my caseload is such that I'll be going to this next review having done nothing in regards to the direct work.
KW: Because of time?
Fiona: Because of time [. . .] so sometimes I'm getting to the point now where I'm tempted to say, 'These children need to be referred to another agency', because acting as a case coordinator is nearly enough. My role with that family at the minute is keeping that placement stable, and keeping mum and the grandparents speaking.

In another interview Enya gives further detail about this issue:

KW: Do you discuss with Emmet [the question] 'Why are you in care?'
Enya: I mean, that's always a difficult area to address with him, and I suppose, you know, it maybe highlights maybe one particular issue about field social workers, not responsibility as such, but the field social worker hasn't time to sit down in a proper format to discuss these issues, you know, because we've tended to do it with other people, which has been either residential social workers, outside agencies or actually the foster carers.

Typical and atypical practice

This chapter has, up until this point, identified the barriers that exist for social workers in terms of building relationships and communicating with young children. It has been argued that the barriers reflect a set of taken-for-granted practices or habits – that we have termed the social worker professional habitus – that has developed over time in response to broader organizational norms and priorities (Ruch 2010a, 2010b). Within this context it is possible to identify typical practices, which have been formed around particular views of young children and issues of risk and harm and that have resulted in distant or non-existent relationships between social workers and young children.

Having said this, there were a few examples from the present research that represented exceptions to the rule and that were characterized by pockets of good social work practice where the importance of relationships with, and the rights of, young children were prioritized. These could be defined as examples of atypical practice. There were two aspects that stood out: first, an emphasis on the competencies of young children; second, an emphasis on the rights of and importance of relationship with young children. The emphasis by this tiny minority of social workers on what young children could do (as opposed to what they could not do) seemed to reflect their newly qualified status, their special interest in direct work with children and their own personal experience of current parenting of young children.

The focus on what young children could do was reflected in Haven's discussion about Harvey. Haven (a newly qualified social worker) seemed genuinely impressed by her observations (and other professionals' observations) of Harvey's level of insight and skills at the age of 4.

Haven: Harvey would be a child who is, he's very, very happy, he's very content, a very joyful insightful child, very animated, very, very, he's so bright, and that was picked up in his pre-adoptive medical, they could not believe how intelligent he was.

KW: How, what kind of things stuck out for them?

Haven: In terms of his assessment, the fact that he, his, his language, his, the way he could form sentences and make stories up and things like that and his understanding of what they were saying, and whenever they were asking him to do particular things he automatically kind of understood what they were requesting.

Likewise Gillian (another newly qualified social worker) does acknowledge that Grady (aged 4 years) was able to express his views and that those views were an understandable reflection of his circumstances.

KW: And for Grady (aged 4 years), do you think that he's [. . .] able to express his wishes and feelings, in terms of his potential to be involved in decisions?

Gillian: I think he's able to express his wishes and feelings. I think he is able, I mean he would clearly say he, he wants to go home to mummy but on the other hand he would say 'no' he wants to stay with Gwendolyn [foster carer]. So I think Grady is going to be a child that you're going to have divided loyalties [. . .] because he really loves his mummy [. . .] and she loves him and [. . .] he wants to be [near her] but he is also pulled towards Gwendolyn.

These examples indicate that some social workers saw and appreciated young children's competencies and their participatory potential within the context of relationships. These social workers identified young children's insight, intelligence and verbal communication skills. In another example, a team manager reflected on the practice of two of her colleagues who were both new to the team where they prioritized, in their daily practice, the rights of and relationships with young children.

KW: And what makes [Jess] stand out, what is it about her?

Joyce: The children are first and foremost, it's what the children think, what the children need, if the children's behaviours are enough to send me squealing out a building Jess will stick with them. I only discovered yesterday she's doing contact with them all on Sunday! That's typical of her, right, they need to have contact with their siblings, they're all over the country, the sooner Jess can do it, it's so important for them to know for their sense of identity and their sense of [*does not finish sentence*].

KW: And is that an unusual approach, do you think?

Joyce: I think it is a bit, I found her refreshing in her work with kids, I have to say, and we've got a new guy here now too, Julian, he was talking about being introduced to a family that he's taken over from somebody else, and there's a very difficult, very disturbed 11-year-old. I said, 'Are you going to meet him?' He says, 'Well, I thought I might meet him out of the house'. 'That's OK', I says, 'Are you going to bring him up here?' and he says, 'No, I was going to take him out to play football'. I said, 'Football? Good God! You are so busy, you're going to play football?' and it was only afterwards and I thought about it and I thought, 'That is a really good idea. Go and do that, go and play football with him. If he agrees to do that with you, that's progress'.

As well as length of qualification, it seems that personal experience made a difference as to how social workers understood relationships with young children:

KW: In your opinion, is there an age at which children shouldn't be part of decision-making processes?

Enya: I suppose that's a tough one because it, I mean, children, being a parent myself, you know, you can see that children obviously develop and mature at different stages in their lives [. . .] I'm of the opinion that all children in some way or other will communicate with you about being in care and I say a child as young as 1 in that [. . .] I do believe that children as young as 1 can tell us about being in care and it takes an experienced and skilled worker to recognize that [. . .] I think that there are things that you need to look for and there are things that you can learn from very young children who tend to, who can easily be forgotten about within the system.

In the present research these atypical attitudes and practices, far from being openly accepted within existing social work teams, appeared to upset the 'status quo' (this is the way we do things) and therefore draw attention to the existing practice norms where children were not viewed as having high levels of competence and where relationships with them were not always viewed as a priority. An example of this upset to the status quo is illustrated by Gillian who discussed her team's reaction to newly introduced practices.

A new chair of the 'children in care' review meetings (LAC meetings) was encouraging children's attendance at their meetings. A series of practical new measures included building up a relationship with each child prior to the meeting by visiting them at their homes, as well as other measures as seen in the example below. Initially the practices of Gloria (the new chair) were not well received by social work colleagues:

Gillian: Gloria [the chair] [. . .] would've started this bringing in cartons of juice and sweets to meetings and sort of she was sort of laughed at in the beginning you know, 'what are you doing?'

KW: [*Later in the interview*] So she's doing that for the children who are coming into their meetings?

Gillian: Yeah. Out of her own pocket!

KW: [*Later in interview*] Why, why would people have laughed at her?

Gillian: I think people just thought, 'oh this is a meeting, this is a meeting you know this is a meeting, what are you doing this for?' because that's the way we looked at LACs.

KW: Do you think it fine-tunes the focus back onto the child?

Gillian: Yeah it can do yeah, I mean I think we were just so dumbfounded, you know 'what, what is she doing?' But I think you know, she had it, you know she'd worked out what she was doing. We are family and childcare but we have no provision for children being in the office. You know and that's, that's quite disturbing.

Because Gloria continued with this practice, regardless of its initial reception by colleagues, it began to act as a catalyst for change. It made social workers reflect on their own professional practices that hindered relationships with young children. Over a period of time Gillian said that individual social workers' practices were reshaped and also led to broader organizational change with the introduction of new local practical guidelines.

Many of the barriers identified in this chapter are being addressed by the government in England through its implementation plan (DCSF 2010a) that outlines how it intends to follow through on the recommendations for reform made by the Social Work Task Force in 2009 (DCSF 2009c, 2009d). A Social Work Reform Board has been established to oversee the process. Significantly, for social workers already in post, a new national standard will be agreed and implemented regarding what support social workers should expect from their employers to do their job effectively. This standard will include attention to training, time and tools.

Summary

This chapter has been concerned with outlining and understanding the social work professional habitus. As explained, the habitus reflects the taken-for-granted practices – or habits – of social workers that they tend to form in response to the pressures of the broader organizational context of the social work profession. In this chapter we have focused on attempting to identify those elements of the social work professional habitus that have tended to inhibit the building of meaningful relationships with children.

More specifically, we have considered seven core barriers – namely, tasks, trust, threats, theories, training, tools and time. It has been shown that these have a significant impact on social workers' ability to build meaningful relationships and to communicate with young children.

However, the chapter has also shown that these barriers are not typical, in their entirety, of all social work practice and nor do they exist uniformly across all individual practice. Indeed, there are examples of social work practice that are characterized more by an emphasis on children's rights and children's competencies. As we have seen, this alternative emphasis creates the right climate for social worker relationships with young children to flourish. The next chapter builds on these alternative ways of doing and thinking, with their emphasis on children's rights and children's competencies, and outlines a framework for practice that would help both social work organizations and social workers revisit their assumptions and values about young children, rethink their methods and revitalize their practices.

4 A child rights-based approach

Summary of chapter content

The purpose of this chapter is to highlight that in order to address the barriers in social workers' relationships with young children, and to compliment the process of reform currently underway, the UNCRC should be explicitly adopted as the guiding framework from which a set of detailed practice guidelines can be drawn up and implemented to help improve practice in building relationships and communicating with young children. In particular, the chapter highlights the principles of the UNCRC and their centrality to effective social work with young children before concluding with a framework of best practice principles that can be used as both a set of guidelines for daily practice and an audit tool.

Introduction

> We believe that the greatest gains in reforming our care system are to be made in identifying and removing whatever barriers are obstructing the development of good personal relationships, and putting in place all possible means of supporting such relationships where they occur.
>
> (HC CSF 2009: 27)

As noted in Chapters One and Two, the social work profession is undergoing a period of significant reform in the light of the high-profile deaths of Victoria Climbié and Peter Connelly and the weaknesses in practice exposed in the subsequent inquiries and progress reports (Laming 2003, 2009). The task of reforming the social work profession is complex given the many organizational and individual practice factors, which, as noted in Chapter Three, can deter social workers from relating to and communicating with young children. As a result, the actual reform process has several key aims but, within this, and influenced by all of the inquiries, there is an emphasis on improving relationships. The recently published House of Commons Children, Schools and Families Select Committee report acknowledges this and also recognizes that change is required at both the organizational and the individual level when it states:

> How can a large bureaucracy possibly act towards individual children in a way that simulates the personal care and attention of a mother or father? Relationships

are extremely difficult to influence directly, and it cannot simply be mandated from the centre that all children have access to someone they can trust, who listens to them and who manifestly cares about them. The only way that the state can hope to achieve this is by empowering the individuals who are responsible for decisions, or present in a child's life, on a daily basis.

(HC CSF 2009: 27)

This chapter argues that, as part of the proposed reforms, there should be new practice guidelines regarding social work with children that should be *explicitly* and *fully* based on the principles of the UNCRC (UN 1989). Currently the focus of reforms is on the structure of social work services, social work training and issues regarding social work governance, accountability and inter-agency cooperation. This chapter argues that, alongside all of this, there is a need for social worker relationships with children to reflect a child rights-based approach through the explicit and full adoption of the UNCRC as a framework from which detailed practice guidelines can be drawn up. It will be argued that this is important because fundamentally what the UNCRC does is to capture the vision of the child as a person, as an individual of worth and as someone to be treated with dignity and respect.

It will be seen that this approach to the child encourages a response that sees beyond the child as a 'case' and instead sees the child as a person able to make contributions to relationships as well as to receive compassion and concern in the course of their relationships with others, including social workers. This focus on the child as a person demands that social workers conduct their relationships with children differently. It means that social workers start from the assumption that children can engage in meaningful relationships with us (rather than the assumption that they cannot do this). It means that social workers start from the assumption that all children, regardless of their age, can express their views and that these views might be expressed in a variety of ways other than just verbally or in writing. Reflective of this framework, it also requires social workers to ask questions such as, 'What does the world look like through your eyes?' 'What is it like to be in your shoes?' 'How best can I help you connect with me to share with me what your experiences and feelings are?' These changes might appear subtle but they reflect a more fundamental shift in thinking about the value and importance social workers attach to children and their relationships with them and how they go about communicating with young children in practice.

O'Neill (2008) reminds us that it is not an option to adopt the principles of the UNCRC, but rather it is a legal requirement. O'Neill also points out that for an organization, and the individuals within it, to fully reflect a child rights-based approach several stages in that transformation have to be completed. First, everyone has to be familiar with the UNCRC and its principles. Second, an analysis is required into what rights are potentially being breached by what practices. Third, a process of capacity-building is required to enable those responsible for fulfilling children's rights (in this case, social work organizations) to honour those rights and for those claiming their rights (in this case, children) to be enabled to lay claim to their rights.

With all this is mind the chapter considers in more detail the remit and function of the United Nations and the principles of the UNCRC. The chapter then applies these principles to case examples from the child abuse inquiries outlined in Chapter One to show how and in what ways children's rights have been breached. The chapter then concludes with an exploration of what practical steps could be taken to improve practice in terms of building relationships and communicating with young children.

The United Nations and the UNCRC

The United Nations (UN) was founded in 1945. Every country belongs to it and it aims to promote international peace and security as well as develop better living standards and contribute to social progress globally. The UN considers and takes action on many issues and particularly on the development of international and national human rights law. While the UN is clear that human rights apply to all age groups, children have received special attention given their age, vulnerability and their need for care and protection. This view is supported internationally and has helped pave the way for the emergence of the UNCRC – the United Nations Convention on the Rights of the Child.

The UNCRC was adopted by the United Nations General Assembly in 1989. The UNCRC defines a child as anyone whose age is anywhere from birth up to the age of 18 years. The UNCRC views children as individuals entitled to a range of basic rights and freedoms and as active contributors exercising these rights within the context of their families and their community. The UNCRC upholds the value, dignity and worth of each and every child and states of childhood:

> [T]he child, by reason of his [or her] physical and mental immaturity, needs special safeguards and care, including appropriate legal protection.
>
> (UN 1989: Preamble)

The UNCRC has four main principles:

- That all children should be free from all forms of discrimination (article 2).
- That in all plans and decision-making affecting the child their best interests are a primary consideration (article 3).
- That all children have the inherent right to life, survival and development (article 6).
- That all children have the right to express their views and for those views to be taken seriously (article 12).

As outlined in Chapter Two, the UNCRC also defines children's provision, protection and participation rights. All of the articles of the UNCRC, which are summarized in Table 4.1, are indivisible and interdependent. This means that they cannot be considered in isolation from each other but that the achievement of any particular right is dependent on the successful implementation of the others. Furthermore, the rights they define are not contingent on what children do or on children's responsibilities.

With regard to Table 4.1, it is important to note that, while summary tables like this are useful, one of the problems has been that people do not read the original version of the UNCRC. In not reading the original version much is missed of the detailed articles outlining the provision, participation and protection rights of all children. Social workers are, therefore, strongly urged to take time to read the UNCRC directly and in its entirety.

The UNCRC is aimed at, and places obligations on, governments and the various organizations and agencies of government that it collectively terms 'state parties'. This

Table 4.1 Types of rights in the UNCRC and supporting articles

Rights in the UNCRC	Supporting articles
Protection Rights	• Protection from kidnapping (article 11) • Protection from all forms of violence, abuse, neglect and discrimination (articles 2 and 19) • Protection of particular groups of children including those without a family, refugees and children with disabilities (articles 20–23 and 32)
Provision Rights	• Provision of services that conform to acceptable standards (article 3) • Provision for health (article 24) • Provision for social security (article 26) • Provision for standard of living (article 27) • Provision for education (articles 28 and 29) • Provision of guidance, information and support (articles 13 and 40)
Participation Rights	• Right to express views freely, to have these taken into account (article 12) • Right to receive and impart information in a media of the child's choice (article 13) • Right to be represented in all decisions made about them and right to freedom of thought, conscience and/or religion (articles 14–17) • Right to participate in arts, culture, leisure and play activities (articles 30, 31)

includes social services departments and thus the standards contained in the UNCRC are directly applicable to social workers. In this sense, social workers, along with all of those who work for the government, are what are termed 'duty bearers' and the UNCRC places a responsibility on them for ensuring that everyone who provides and cares for children knows about and is guided by the provisions contained in the UNCRC (article 42). In a similar way, alongside those working for government are duty bearers in the context of the UNCRC, children are considered to be 'rights holders' (O'Neill 2008).

EXERCISE
Before reading on, complete the following:

• Read through the UNCRC and identify articles that are relevant to social work practice with young children known to social services.
• Consider ways in which the articles you have selected are indivisible and interdependent.

The UNCRC and social work law, policy and practice

It is already the case, as recently summarized by the government in a draft report (DCSF Children's Rights and Participation Team 2010) that government legislation concerning children and social work reflects parts of the UNCRC in its statutory duties to protect, provide for, listen to and respect children (Children Act 1989, The Children (Northern Ireland) Order 1995; Children (Scotland) Act 1995; Children Act 2004; Childcare Act 2006; Children and Young Persons Act 2008). In Northern Ireland, Scotland and Wales there are active children's rights commissioners but in England the role of the children's commissioner is more constrained being tasked with 'having regard to' the UNCRC and not actively promoting it as the other commissioners do.

Furthermore, government policies about social work and children do make reference to the importance of the UNCRC as a set of guiding principles. As noted in Chapter One, there are three groups of children known to social services: those at risk of harm, those in need of support and those in care. For children at risk of harm the statutory guidance *Working Together to Safeguard Children* (DCSF 2010b) states that the document is underpinned by the principles of the UNCRC and that these should be reflected in day-to-day practice, but, having said this, it does not provide a framework illustrating specifically how and in what ways the new guidelines map onto and/or reflect the principles of the UNCRC. For children in need of support the guidance accompanying the Common Assessment Framework also claims to be underpinned by principles of empowerment and inclusivity reflective of a child rights framework (CWDC 2009: 23).

In addition the non-statutory guidance *Common Core of Skills and Knowledge for the Children's Workforce* (DfES 2005) also mentions the UNCRC. This particular set of guidelines was recently reviewed and one issue to be considered was whether the UNCRC should be more explicitly incorporated. As it stands, the UNCRC is only referenced in passing. More specifically, in the updated 'Common Core' guidelines (CWDC 2010), while in evidence indirectly through the recommendations for improvement, children's rights are explicitly mentioned just once and this is in general terms, as noted, when the document states that '[t]he common core acknowledges the rights of children and young people, and the role parents, carers and families play in helping achieve positive outcomes' (CWDC 2010: 12). As we will see in this chapter, an opportunity has therefore been missed here to begin with the UNCRC and the associated General Comments and to use them as the basic framework from which to develop practice principles. This compares with the *Care Matters* policy agenda in England, Wales and Northern Ireland that explicitly references the UNCRC.

Lastly, there are also practice developments, in the form of guides by voluntary organizations, local social work departments and government bodies (VCC/NCB 2004; NCB 2006) that are designed specifically to further develop knowledge, skills and values in relation to social work with children and that do make reference to the UNCRC.

The UN Committee, that oversees the implementation of the UNCRC, remains concerned that the government, at times, pays 'lip service' to children's rights and has not done enough to fully implement the UNCRC in law, policy and practice. In their latest report the UN Committee urges the UK government to

> further strengthen its efforts to ensure that all of the provisions of the Convention are widely known and understood by adults [and to reinforce these with] adequate and systematic training of all professional groups working for and with children, in particular law enforcement officials, immigration officials, media, teachers, health personnel, social workers and personnel of childcare institutions.
>
> (UN 2008: 5, para. 21)

Furthermore, research shows that, in day-to-day social work practice there is little awareness of the UNCRC. In England, for example, the Children's Rights Alliance for England (CRAE 2009) reported that a major barrier to the realization of children's rights is social workers' lack of knowledge about the UNCRC. In its written submission to the then government's Children, Schools and Families Select Committee, CRAE highlighted the need for systematic training on the UNCRC for all professionals working with and for children (CRAE 2009). Kilkelly *et al.* (2004) and Scottish Alliance for Children's Rights (SACR 2009) report similar findings and recommendations regarding the status of children's rights in Northern Ireland and Scotland.

In order to highlight how the framework could better inform and shape social work practice the chapter highlights, through revisiting some of the findings of the child abuse inquiries outlined in Chapter One, what social work practices have breached the UNCRC principles and then considers how the UNCRC could be used as a framework to inform and shape future social work childcare practice. In doing this, the chapter also takes account of a number of the General Comments published by the UN Committee on specific issues connected to the interpretation and implementation of certain articles of the UNCRC. There are 12 General Comments and, in this chapter, No. 5 (*General Measures of Implementation*) (UN 2003), No. 7 *Implementing Child Rights in Early Childhood*) (UN 2005), No. 9 (*The Rights of Children with Disabilities*) and No. 12 (*The Right of the Child to be Heard*) (UN 2009) have particular relevance for social work.

Social work practice and breaches of children's rights

What does it mean to breach children's rights? What exactly does this look like in practice? What is the consequence for the child or the impact on the child of breaches of their rights? A way of helping social workers answer these questions is to apply the principles and provisions to case examples. Below, the four founding principles of the UNCRC – non-discrimination (article 2); best interests (article 3); the right to be heard (article 12); and the right to life, survival and development (article 6) – are applied to a number of child abuse inquiries to help inform social workers' understanding of the way in which specific rights can and have been breached in social work practice with young children. From this it is possible to consider how and in what ways the UNCRC might inform and shape more effective practice in terms of building relationships and communicating with young children.

Non-discrimination

Under article 2 of the UNCRC, governments and their agencies are under an obligation to protect children from discrimination. In particular, the UNCRC states that governments:

1   Shall respect and ensure the rights [of children] without discrimination of any kind, irrespective of the child's or his or her parent's or legal guardian's race, colour, sex, language, religion, political or other opinion, national, ethnic or social origin, property, disability, birth or other status.
2   Shall take all appropriate measures to ensure that the child is protected against all forms of discrimination or punishment on the basis of the status, activities, expressed opinions, or beliefs of the child's parents, legal guardians, or family members.

While the UNCRC omits discrimination on the basis of age, subsequent General

Comments No. 7 and No. 12 (UN 2005, UN 2009) have made particular comment on this. For example, General Comment No. 7 states:

> Article 2 means that young children in general must not be discriminated against on any grounds [. . .] Young children are especially at risk of discrimination because they are relatively powerless and depend on others for the realisation of their rights.
>
> (UN 2005: 5, para. 11)

In the case of Victoria Climbié, who was originally from the Ivory Coast in Africa and had moved to England with her aunt, social workers' assumptions about her colour and culture closed down opportunities for them to understand Victoria's life from her point of view (Laming 2003: 345–7, paras 16.1–13; Welbourne 2002). For example, Victoria's relationship with her carers was described as a 'master/servant' relationship (Laming 2003: 148, para. 6.220) and this was assumed to relate to Ivory Coast traditions in parenting and childhood deference and respect towards elders (Laming 2003: 150, para. 6.232). No one explored with Victoria why she was anxious in the presence of her carers, why she felt it necessary to stand to attention in their presence or why on several occasions, when being visited by her carers in hospital, she wet herself (Laming 2003: 234, para. 8.75).

Although the report of the Laming Inquiry into the circumstances regarding the death of Victoria Climbié (2003) does not directly reference article 2 (UN 1989) Laming's comments do reflect its content. He says that

> [t]he basic requirement that children are kept safe is universal and cuts across cultural boundaries. Every child living in this country is entitled to be given the protection of the law, regardless of his or her background. [. . .] Every organisation concerned with the welfare and protection of children should have mechanisms in place to ensure equal access to services of the same quality, and that each child, irrespective of colour or background, should be treated as an individual requiring appropriate care.
>
> (Laming 2003: 346, para. 16.10)

In this instance, social workers' prejudices and assumptions about the family's norms based on the family's cultural background, in the words of Laming (2003: 345, para. 16.3), 'diverted caring people from noting and acting upon signs of neglect or ill-treatment'. For example, in Victoria's case, assumptions based on a particular concept of the Afro-Caribbean family clouded social workers' judgements about issues of neglect and abuse. Laming points out how the social worker said in the inquiry of Victoria 'standing to attention' before Ms Kouao and Mr Manning 'that this type of relationship was one that can be seen in many Afro-Caribbean families because respect and obedience are very important features of the Afro-Caribbean family script' (Laming 2003: 345, para. 16.4). He went on to say, in the same paragraph, that 'Victoria's parents, however, made it clear that she was not required to stand in this formal way when she was at home with them. Therefore it seems [the social worker's] assumption was unfounded, in Victoria's case at least'. The Laming report provides this and other similar evidence to show how social workers' assumptions and prejudices discriminated against Victoria in that she was denied protection against harm on the basis of culture and race. Partly as a result of this her needs were never properly assessed and her protection rights were not properly afforded her.

Alongside discrimination on the basis of culture and/or race, it is clear from many of the inquiry reports that the children were discriminated against on the basis of their age. Although never explicitly explored in the inquiries into the deaths of Maria Colwell, Jasmine Beckford, Peter Connelly and other young children, it seems that part of the failure to listen to children was related to age-related discrimination and assumptions about children's capacity to express their views. As noted earlier, General Comment No. 7 warns against 'discrimination [that] may take the form of [. . .] inhibition of free expression of feelings and views' (UN 2005: 5, para. 11(b)).

Peter Connelly is particularly relevant here. He was called 'Baby P' and, in the media, computer generated images of a 6- to 8-month-old baby were used to show where his body was injured. And yet Peter Connelly was a 17-month-old toddler – walking, talking and capable of sophisticated exchanges in his relationships. An important point for social workers to note, and one that we will return to later, is that social context, life experience, development, abilities and personalities of the children all influence children's capacities (Alderson 2000/2008). On this point the UN Committee also states:

> Respect for the young child's agency – as a participant in family, community and society – is frequently overlooked, or rejected on the grounds of age and immaturity [. . .]. They have been regarded as undeveloped, lacking even basic capacities for understanding, communicating and making choices. They have been powerless within their families, and often voiceless and invisible within society. The Committee wishes to emphasize that article 12 applies both to younger and to older children [. . .]. Young children [. . .] make choices and communicate their feelings, ideas and wishes in numerous ways, long before they are able to communicate through the conventions of spoken or written language.
>
> (UN 2005: 6–7, para. 14)

Best interests

The best interests principle is already enshrined in childcare legislation and appears in a number of UNCRC articles – namely, articles 9, 18, 20 and 21 (UN 1989). Most commonly it is quoted as article 3 that states:

> In all actions concerning children, whether undertaken by public or private social welfare institutions, courts of law, administrative authorities or legislative bodies, the best interests of the child shall be a primary consideration.
>
> (UN 1989: 2)

For social workers the best interests principle is most commonly experienced as the tension between what adults determine to be in the best interests of the child (article 3) as compared with children's own divergent wishes and feelings (article 12). It is also mistakenly played out in practice as being what adults determine to be best for children without consultation with the child. However, the UN Committee makes clear that it is not possible to come to a decision about a child's best interests without consulting the child. In particular, and reflecting the principle of the indivisibility of rights as outlined earlier, the Committee states:

There is no tension between articles 3 and 12, only a complimentary role of the two general principles: one establishes the objective of achieving the best interests of the child and the other provides the methodology for reaching the goal of hearing either the child or the children. In fact, there can be no correct application of article 3 if the components of article 12 are not respected. Likewise, article 3 reinforces the functionality of article 12, facilitating the essential role of children in all decisions affecting their lives.

(UN 2009: 15–6, paras 71, 74)

Integral, therefore, to the *process* of determining the best interests of the child is respect for other rights, particularly article 12 that specifies the right of the child to form and express views. This is a clear example of the indivisibility and interdependence of children's rights as defined within the UNCRC. Even pre-verbal children can express fear or confidence, affection or mistrust vividly in their body language, and the body itself graphically records and expresses children's experiences – for example, of injury. If adults' decisions are to be informed they have to take as much account as possible of the children's views. Inquiry reports show that the best interests principle found in article 3 was breached because in the cases of Maria Colwell, Peter Connelly ('Baby P') and Jasmine Beckford professionals made decisions about what they thought was in the best interests of the children (either keeping them with their parents or returning them to their parents) without reference to the children's own wishes and feelings.

Right to be heard

In social work, probably the best-known and most frequently quoted UNCRC article is that of children's right to express their views (article 12). This article states:

1 States Parties shall assure to the child who is capable of forming his or her own views the right to express those views freely in all matters affecting the child, the views of the child being given due weight in accordance with the age and maturity of the child.
2 For this purpose, the child shall in particular be provided the opportunity to be heard in any judicial and administrative proceedings affecting the child, either directly, or through a representative or an appropriate body, in a manner consistent with the procedural rules of national law.

(UN 1989: 4)

The process of facilitating young children's participation rights therefore depends on the information given (UNCRC article 13, 42), the child's own experiences and capacities (article 5), the wider societal expectations and norms (article 5, 14 and 42) and the level of support available. The UN Committee has recently highlighted these components of the participation process when it states:

Children's levels of understanding are not uniformly linked to their biological age. Research has shown that information, experience, environment, social and cultural expectations, and levels of support all contribute to the development of a child's capacities to form a view.

(UN 2009: 8, para. 29)

As we have also seen earlier, inquiry reports provide many examples of how social workers breached children's rights to express their views freely in all of these areas and how making best interests decisions was compromised. For example, and as indicated in Chapter One, Maria Colwell's views about the plan to return her home were simply ignored. She had strongly indicated her disagreement at the plan to return her home through her behaviour. However, the social worker did not actively explore with Maria her views, the reasons underpinning her behaviour, or refer her to someone more specialized, but instead made a series of assumptions and guesses. Having minimized the behaviour and, in effect, silenced Maria's own voice, the plan towards rehabilitation was pursued in spite of Maria's protests. Furthermore, Maria was not provided with information about the date and manner of her return home. Instead, on the day of the planned return and as also noted in Chapter One, her birth mother told Maria that she was only visiting for the weekend and that she would see her main carers in a few days. This was a lie with which the social worker (who was present) actively colluded and, as noted in Chapter One, Maria was never to see her main carers of seven years ever again.

With regard to Victoria Climbié, the Laming report into her death (Laming 2003) provides evidence of how Victoria's rights were breached under a number of articles. These included articles 2, 5, 12–14 and 42. This can be seen, for example, in the hospital social worker's failure to talk with Victoria, enlist an interpreter to engage Victoria in the initial assessment process, or seek her views in the investigation of abuse for fear of contaminating evidence (Laming 2003, p. 237–8, para. 8.97). The Laming report notes that these practices were shared by a number of professionals. Again while not referencing the UNCRC directly Laming does underline the importance of seeking the views of children when he states that

> [s]eeing, listening to and observing the child must be an essential element of an initial assessment for any social worker [and that, in this case, the role of the social worker was] simply to listen [to Victoria] without interruption and to record and evaluate what has been said.
>
> (Laming 2003: 238, para. 8.99)

Right to life, survival and development

Inquiries show that the lack of meaningful relationship was one factor that led to breaches of other rights, particularly the children's right to be protected from abuse (articles 19, 34, 37) and their right to life, survival and development (article 6). Article 6 states:

1 States Parties recognize that every child has the inherent right to life.
2 States Parties shall ensure to the maximum extent possible the survival and development of the child.

On this principle, and in relation to young children, the UN Committee reminds us that

> [e]nsuring survival and physical health are priorities. [However,] article 6 encompasses all aspects of development [and these rights] can only be implemented in a

holistic manner with attention to all areas of a child's development and the early involvement of children in paying attention to their own well being.

(UN 2005: 4, para. 10)

The child abuse inquiries show how their survival rights were breached through a failure to attend to all aspects of the children's development and well-being in a holistic manner. For example, all of the inquiries note poor inter-agency cooperation and information-sharing that had the consequence of increasing the risk that children's rights were breached.

Developing a rights-based approach

So far, the principles of the UNCRC have been explored and applied in case examples to illustrate how and in what ways social workers, through their poor relationships with children, have breached children's rights. This section considers what a rights-based approach might look like and how it could lead to better relationships and more effective communication between social workers and young children.

The serious case review into the death of Peter Connelly speaks of the need for social workers to adopt the right 'mode of relationship' with the parents (Haringey LSCB 2009: 25). What we have to think about is what is the right 'mode of relationship' between social workers and the children known to them? As noted in earlier chapters and in the light of the *Care Matters* policy agenda (DfES 2006, 2007), recent reports from Laming (Laming 2003, 2009), the House of Commons Children, Schools and Families Select Committee (HC CSF 2009) and the implementation of the Children and Young Persons Act 2008, there are new models of practice that have been introduced and are being piloted with the aim of putting the social worker–child relationship back at the centre of effective practice. These new structures, which include, among others, social work practices and social pedagogical approaches to the delivery of care in the residential sector, are currently being evaluated to see whether they are successful in their aim of securing better outcomes for children through social workers (and other professionals) developing positive, consistent and meaningful relationships with children.

However, as seen by the recent cases of Victoria and Peter (and the many others that have not made the headlines) policy and practice improvements are urgently required in terms of social workers building meaningful relationships and communicating with young children. In this regard, the UNCRC and associated General Comments provide the best framework for improving practice and training because, as stated earlier, they: offer a definition of the child as of individual worth, value, a rights bearer and an active contributor (as opposed to passive recipient) from the earliest age; provide detailed guidance to help challenge some of the key stumbling blocks in day-to-day practice in terms of children's capacity, the free expression of views, giving views due weight according to the child's age and maturity; and they provide a framework for implementation with detailed guidance provided in General Comment No. 5 (UN 2003). Furthermore, it is important to remember that whether these arguments are convincing or not it is, ultimately, immaterial because the government is obliged by international law to implement the UNCRC and that therefore includes its provision of social work services. In light of these arguments and the legal requirement to do so the specific contribution of the UNCRC is now considered under the headings of social work values, knowledge and skills.

Social worker values

It is of vital importance that social workers have self-knowledge in relation to their own attitudes and assumptions regarding young children because, as seen through the interviews with social workers in Chapter Three, these have an impact on whether and how they form relationships and communicate with young children. Most adults hold a range of attitudes and assumptions towards young children that may also be contradictory and ambiguous. Aside from their variety, another difficulty is that they often represent the professional habitus or social workers' unconscious, unspoken and taken-for-granted ways of thinking. According to Alderson (2000/2008), who has also undertaken pioneering research with young children regarding their perspectives on their life-limiting illnesses (Alderson 1993), two things have to happen to bring hidden assumptions and attitudes from the unconscious into the conscious: first, there is a need to name them; second, to then try to work out the belief system from which they emanate.

In practice with young children under the age of 8 years, social workers are used to viewing young children as clients and/or in need of care and/or control. They are less used to viewing young children as individuals with their own contributions to make to assessment and decision-making processes. As illustrated through the interviews with social workers in Chapter Three, this inevitably affects the relationships they develop with young children. Children are not approached as individuals but rather there is a tendency to disbelieve that they have valuable contributions to make or that they are reliable, trustworthy and competent.

Social workers need to begin the process of changing their practice by rethinking their own values and assumptions about young children. By embedding the UNCRC in training and practice guidelines social workers would first have to acknowledge practice that reflected discriminatory age-related assumptions about children and their abilities (UN 1989 article 2, UN 2005, UN 2009). Second, and related to this, they need to start from the premise that a child does have the capacity to form his or her views, that they have a right to express those views and that it is not up to the child to first prove their capacity (UN 2009: 6, para. 20).

How can social workers actually address in practice their assumptions and values towards young children? Practical ways of achieving this are described in detail in Chapters Five and Six. However, and as a general principle, there is no substitute for spending time with young children in order to gain insight into their competencies and capacities. It is one thing reading in a book that social workers should value all children and their contributions; it is another seeing this in reality. Spending time with young children would reveal that their interaction and communication, far from being just 'child's play', is actually nuanced, insightful and meaningful. It is frightening to think that social workers can qualify to work in child protection without any experience of direct contact with young children. Social work training for family and childcare social workers should, therefore, involve mandatory placements with young children in nursery and pre-school settings in order to see, learn, receive and experience the skills that young children bring to their relationships with those around them. This would undoubtedly change attitudes and assumptions as well as the taken-for-granted working knowledge that social workers have about children, childhood and children's development.

Social worker knowledge

As we have seen in Chapter Two, social workers have been criticized for not knowing enough about how children develop, not knowing how to read and interpret children's behaviour, not knowing what the signs and symptoms of abuse are and of not knowing how to communicate with young children. Olive Stevenson, an eminent professor in social work, reflecting on the Jasmine Beckford inquiry suggested that the social worker's relationship with Jasmine suffered because of a lack of a clear theoretical underpinning in terms of children's development and children's behaviour. She stated that

> [p]erhaps the most crucial issue of all [. . .] is the failure of the social worker to observe, assess and communicate effectively with children. [The] skills of relating to such children and making use of the information still lag behind in social work practice. [. . .] As social work has reacted against too uncritical an espousal of psychodynamic theory, as it has sought explanations of behaviour from a social structural perspective, it has left its students singularly ill-equipped to deal with confused, ambivalent, uncertain messages from troubled children at home. What, for example, are the quiet children like Maria and Jasmine seeking to convey? Are they withdrawn and depressed or are they just quiet? What are the messages of drawings, play, actions rather than words? These are some of the matters that have to be addressed in the changed climate of social work education if social workers are to protect children more effectively than Maria and Jasmine were protected. If psychodynamic theory is no longer to be used as a basis for such understanding, what alternative theoretical frameworks are we offering?
>
> (Stevenson 1986: 506–7)

Stevenson's comments draw attention to the necessity of social workers being equipped with appropriate theoretical knowledge about children and their development. As argued already, some of this knowledge will come from practice and direct contact with young children while other knowledge will be informed by texts. While there is no space in the context of this book to outline the specific and wide-ranging theoretical knowledge in detail (as noted earlier this is done in detail elsewhere, particularly in the work of Trevithick (2005), Aldgate *et al.* (2006) and Horwath (2009)), it is important to reiterate that social workers must be aware of the broad tenets of psychodynamic theory and that they must have knowledge of children's development and its relationship to broader social contexts.

A good illustrative example regarding the importance of theoretical knowledge is the current assessment formats, discussed in earlier chapters, which are theoretically informed by the developmental 'ecological model' (Aldgate *et al.* 2006) that combines the work of Jean Piaget and Urie Bronfenbrenner. This framework helps social workers understand how children's development may be compromised by adversity, challenges and changes in their wider social context. For example, there is research as detailed in Aldgate *et al.* (2006) that shows that young children's exposure to poverty, abuse, neglect, violence, loss, separation, rejection and trauma can have a detrimental impact on their short- and long-term development. Some of the consequences for young children can include behaviours and reactions such as childhood depression, eating disorders and other self-harming behaviours, relationship difficulties, poor educational attainment and poor self-concept, to name but a few and as explored in detail in the work of Aldgate *et al.* (2006).

On the other hand, this framework (and other frameworks such as those on resilience) also illustrate that some young children who have had adverse experiences adapt well and experience few (if any) long-term adverse developmental outcomes. Of equal importance, therefore, are those resilience frameworks that help explain how some young children survive negative experiences better than others by drawing on their own internal strengths as well as strengths in their networks including relationships with significant people, places and pets, for example. The literature on these issues is vast but indicates that some young children's social skills and social competence may be highly developed (Gilligan 2001).

Theoretical and practical knowledge of young children's skills and competence is an important and yet underdeveloped area of social work with young children where more practice and training knowledge is required. One of the criticisms of social workers' relationships with young children has been an over-reliance on rigidly applied age-related schedules that have a tendency to underestimate what young children can do. There is now a substantial body of research that explores young children's competence and illustrates how it is not necessarily age-related (Alderson 1993; Lansdown 2005a, 2005b; Alderson and Morrow 2010). As Alderson (1993: 158) argues,

> [childhood] competence is more influenced by the social context and the child's experience than by innate ability and to respect children means we must not think in sharp dichotomies of wise adult/immature child, infallible doctor/ignorant patient, but to see wisdom and uncertainty shared among people of varying ages and experiences.

These ideas are embedded in the UNCRC through the concept of 'evolving capacities' found in article 5 (UN 1989). In UN General Comment No. 7 (UN 2005) the notion of 'evolving capacities' is defined as a process of learning and maturation whereby children

> progressively acquire knowledge, competencies and understanding about their rights and how best they can be realized [. . .] While a young child generally requires more guidance than an older child, it is important to take account of individual variations in the capacities of children of the same age and of their ways of reacting to situations.
>
> (UN 2005: 8, para. 18)

The General Comment goes on to challenge the rigid application of an age-related approach to understanding the concept of evolving capacities when it states:

> Evolving capacities should be seen as a positive and enabling process, not an excuse for authoritarian practices that restrict children's autonomy and self-expression and which have traditionally been justified by pointing to children's relative immaturity.
>
> (UN 2005: 8, para. 18)

The challenge to age-related assumptions about young children's competencies is made even more explicit in the work of Lansdown when she states:

> Much of the current thinking in respect of children's developmental capacities is derived from Western child development theories, which rest on a presumption that adulthood is the normative state, with children being in a state of immaturity characterised by irrationality, incompetence, passivity and dependence [. . .] This 'deficit' model of childhood leads to a failure to recognise the extent of children's actual capacities. It means that much of what children are capable of is rendered invisible [. . .] Yet, there is a wealth of evidence to counter the prevailing perception of children as incompetent beings, all passing through a universally and pre-determined process of development.
>
> (Lansdown 2005b: 8–9)

Social work training and practice with young children should, therefore, explicitly reference and provide training around the concept of evolving capacities that also fully embraces a knowledge base about children's development that is not founded on age-related discrimination. In Scotland this is well under way in social work practice with the Getting it Right for Every Child (GIRFEC) policy agenda that is firmly rooted in both a children's rights and childhood resilience model.

One theoretical approach that might help social workers critically engage with the fluid concept of evolving capacities is the sociology of childhood. This approach also emphasizes the contextual nature of childhood competence as well as the contextual nature to understanding childhood more generally. This is best illustrated in the work of Jenks (1982), a leading sociologist, who has argued that

> cross-culturally children vary enormously in terms of their degree of responsibility, the expectations held of them, their level of dependency, need for care, life expectation and more generally the nature of their relationship with adults.
>
> (Jenks 1982: 205)

These ideas were developed in the important work of James and Prout (1997). The relevance of their ideas to social work practice with young children is that they challenge our taken-for-granted assumptions about young children and encourage us to view children as active contributors to their own lives and the lives of those around them while also giving prominence to the perspective of the child.

Social worker skills

Connected with this, there are particular skills that are required to build relationships and communicate with young children. In subsequent chapters these principles and skills will be illustrated through detailed case examples involving children from the current research study who were between the ages of 4 and 7 years. For now the chapter provides an outline and explains how and why the UNCRC provides the best framework for spelling those skills and principles out and encouraging organizations and individuals to make them a reality.

It is difficult to write in abstract form about required skills in building relationships and communicating with young children because what are needed are detailed

Table 4.2 UN best practice principles in working with children (UN 2009)

Practice principles	Meaning
Transparent and informative	Children must be provided with full, accessible, diversity-sensitive and age-appropriate information about their right to express their views freely, the weight to be given to their views and how this participation will take place, its scope, purpose and potential impact.
Voluntary	Children should never be coerced into expressing views against their wishes and they should be informed that they can cease involvement at any stage.
Respectful	Children's views have to be treated with respect. Adults should create opportunities, understand the social and economic context of children's lives and build on good practice.
Relevant	Issues should be of relevance to the children, selected by themselves and allow for children to draw on their knowledge, skills and abilities.
Child-friendly	Environments and methods should be adapted to children's capacities. Adequate time, resources, preparation and support should be made available and sensitive to different cultural backgrounds.
Inclusive	Non-discriminatory and encouraging to marginalized groups of children.
Supported by training	Adults need preparation, skills and support to facilitate children's participation effectively. Adults should be provided with skills in listening, working jointly with children and engaging them effectively in accordance with their evolving capacities.
Safe and sensitive to risk	Adults need to be aware of and minimize the risks posed to some children by virtue of their involvement in decision-making.
Accountable	Children must be informed as to how their views have been interpreted, used and how their views have influenced any outcomes. Monitoring and evaluation of children's participation needs to be undertaken, where possible, with children themselves.

examples of how such skills look in practice. This section is, therefore, just a starting point in terms of simply providing an overview of the required skills as outlined in the UNCRC. Subsequent chapters then explore these skills in action through the use of many case examples.

In summary, the UNCRC outlines adults' obligations to create opportunities for children to freely express their views (article 5 UNCRC, UN 1989). Furthermore, General Comment No. 12 (UN 2009) makes it clear that meaningful relationships underpin the creation of opportunities which include: having the right attitude towards children's capacities; creating conditions that reflect the individuality of each child and that afford the child respect and security; providing the right materials, support and equipment; providing the right kind of information to children as it determines their opportunity to respond; and of having well-developed communication and observation skills 'to tune into the messages that children relay to us either directly or indirectly through a variety of means including play, body language, facial expressions, and drawing and painting' (UN 2009: 7–8).

General Comment No. 12 (UN 2009) also reaffirms the basic practice principles that should underpin relationships and communication with young children. These, as summarized in Table 4.2, outline that all practice is to be transparent and informative, voluntary, respectful, relevant, child-friendly, inclusive, supported by training, safe and sensitive to risk and accountable. This list should underpin all social work practice guidelines about building relationships and communicating with young children. Furthermore, these guidelines should be accompanied by case examples illustrating the guidelines in action, thereby helping to reduce the risk that these become just another set of guidelines that look good on paper but bear little relevance to reality. The following chapters do just that – provide in-depth live case material to illustrate the benefit to young children of the principles of the UNCRC in practice.

Summary

This chapter has outlined the contribution that can be made to new practice frameworks by the explicit use of the UNCRC and associated General Comments. Its four cross-cutting principles – of non-discrimination; best interests; rights to life, survival and development; and the right to be heard – provide the foundations for forming meaningful relationships with young children and for developing better communication with them. Its definition of the protection, provision and participation rights of all children, the indivisibility of these rights and explicit guidance on the full implementation of these rights in the form of General Comments provide the framework from which best practice principles can and should be developed. The issue of what this actually looks like in practice is the focus of the next two chapters.

5 Communicating with young children
Stages and skills

Summary of chapter content

This chapter discusses the application of the principles of the UNCRC to social workers communicating with young children. Using the detailed case example of Aine (aged 7 years) and real-life excerpts of conversations with her, the chapter illustrates the stages of the communication process, the skills required to communicate effectively with young children and the ways in which both are embedded in a child rights approach. Exercises and general pointers for effective practice are also provided.

Introduction

While there are many recent examples of helpful resources regarding general communication skills (Trevithick 2005; Koprowska 2008) and specific resources for communicating with children (Butler and Williamson 1994; Davie *et al.* 1996; Bannister *et al.* 1997; Milner and Carolin 1999/2000; Jones 2003; NCB 2004, 2006; Luckock and Lefevre 2008; McLeod 2008b; Lefevre 2010; SCIE 2010), what is often missing are *real-life and detailed transcripts* of social workers' conversations with *young children (under the age of 8 years)* showing the application of the required knowledge, skills and values in practice. There is thus a danger that the resources that are available remain useful external reminders but, because of a lack of practical examples, there is limited opportunity for them to become embedded in the day-to-day practice of social workers. This and the following chapter seek to fill this gap by using examples from my own research with young children to explore, discuss and draw out general themes and demonstrate some of the ways they can be applied in practice.

In this chapter the focus is on one case study, that of Aine, aged 7 years, to illustrate the stages in the communication process, the skills used and the issues arising during conversations and how these were dealt with. Some readers might find some of the interview excerpts that follow lengthy. However, I have purposely not shortened them because they, in their entirety, represent the actual real-life communication process with Aine and illustrate, in detail, what is possible in terms of building relationships and communicating with young children. Moreover, to shorten them would do a disservice to Aine's own capabilities and to her story. It would also do a disservice to those of you who have never had the opportunity to communicate directly and in detail with young children and for whom this might represent the first occasion you have to get close to experiencing first-hand what happens. Before introducing the stages of communication the chapter begins with an introduction to Aine and her family. Ethical issues relating to the research process in respect of Aine, and all other children featured in this book, are detailed in Chapter Seven.

Background information on Aine

In many ways Aine's circumstances, as will become clear, were similar to those of the children whose deaths provided the focus for official inquiries as outlined in Chapter One. Aine lived with her two younger sisters, older brother and her parents. The family had been known to social services for a number of years. There were a number of concerns about her parents including mental health difficulties, violence in their relationships, alcohol dependency and the vulnerability of Aine's mother, who had been in care as a child herself. Social services had offered the family practical and financial support including provision of day nursery places and home visits by a family support service because of concerns about the physical and emotional neglect of the children, who appeared dirty, unfed and who had been left unsupervised for long periods of time.

According to the professionals, the parents' care of their children seemed to improve and support tailed off. After the birth of their youngest child, Angela, social services again received several referrals from the extended family expressing concerns about the care of the children who, it was alleged, were not being fed and supervised appropriately. Social services and health professionals responded and, while managing to make contact with Aine's mother, often did not get to see the children. Following further referrals, social services visited the family home and, on this occasion, insisted on seeing the children who, according to Aine's mother, were asleep upstairs. The social worker found the two youngest children upstairs in appalling conditions. It was apparent that they had been locked in their bedrooms for hours on end without food and access to a toilet. One child, in hunger, had eaten her own faeces. Mattresses had no bedding and were urine sodden. Faeces covered the floor and the walls as high as the children could stand. Later it became clear that all of the children had endured these conditions over a period of several weeks, if not months.

Aine was separated from her siblings and placed in foster care. Her siblings either went into foster care or residential care. At the time of my research Aine had been living away from home for just over two years. She had remained in face-to-face contact with her siblings and birth parents through contact arrangements supervised by social services. Throughout this period she had remained placed with the same foster carers.

Stages and skills in the communication process

The development of knowledge, skills and values in communicating is a key aspect to social work training (Trevithick 2005; Koprowska 2008; Wilson *et al.* 2008; McLeod 2008b; Luckock and Lefevre 2008; SCIE 2010). In this chapter these are applied specifically to communicating with young children to illustrate their application in practice. This is a crucial aspect to improving social workers' relationships with young children, especially in a context where newly trained social workers feel ill-equipped to undertake this vital work (CWDC 2010).

In essence, the process of communicating – which could involve communicating formally in assessment interviews, court proceedings and meetings or less formally in home visits, for example – consists of three stages: beginnings (getting to know you);,middle (exchange of information) and endings (conclusions) (Wilson *et al.* 2008). The fact that the process can be broken down into three stages should not be taken to mean that the communication process is uncomplicated. Trevithick (2005: 81–5) illustrates the complexities involved in terms of the knowledge and skills required. In this chapter each of these stages will be explored and illustrated through the relationship I developed with Aine. The discussion of each stage begins with the outline of some general principles before showing how these were applied in conversation with Aine.

Beginnings

Good beginnings are essential (Koprowska 2008: 51–2; Wilson *et al.* 2008: 301). Having said that, if a conversation does not start well, the situation is not necessarily irretrievable but it may take longer for a conversation to fully develop. Good beginnings are made up of establishing rapport (Trevithick 2005: 147–8) and creating the right conditions (UN 2009: 7–8, 12 and 17) for communication to occur. To establish rapport means to have created a connection that facilitates confidence and cooperation in verbal and non-verbal communication between the people involved in the conversation. The processes of building a rapport can either be slow and gradual or quite immediate. Social workers will know of those occasions where, within a few minutes of a conversation with someone, it feels like a connection has been formed. They will feel comfortable, at ease, safe, secure and there is often a rhythm and a compatibility in terms of the verbal and non-verbal exchanges that take place. Social workers will also know of those occasions where the process is a lot harder.

Some people believe it is particularly hard to build rapport with a young child because of differences in age, size, ability and experience (Alderson 2000/2008). However, adults can often exaggerate these differences, whereas, in fact, young children might have much more experience than their social worker does of certain situations and they may have developed much better skills than their social workers in relation to those situations. For example, Alderson (1993) found that children's experience of living with complex illnesses had enabled them to develop an expertise in their own condition that was more developed than expected. There is thus more overlap in the skills and abilities between children and adults than is often given credit for. In addition, experience shows that each child is different. As such there are no simple 'blueprints' that can be followed but rather, as will now be outlined, a broader set of guiding principles and processes.

To begin with, and where possible, it is a good idea for the social worker to become a familiar figure by visiting the home, school and/or clubs when the child is there in the few days before they are due to speak with them. While no in-depth communication might take place between the social worker and the child, the child will have seen the social worker in different settings of familiarity to them and a social worker's presence in those settings builds up a bank of shared memories on which the social worker and child can both draw when the meeting does take place. It is worth the social worker therefore taking a note of the different contexts in which they have seen the child so that when they do later meet they have concrete things to talk about. For example, a conversation might begin with the question, 'Do you remember the last time I saw you? You were at the family centre playing with that doll's house with the little bed in it?'

Creating the right conditions, as noted in the previous chapter, involves a number of things including: having the right attitude towards children's capacities; respecting the individuality of each child; affording the child security; providing the right materials, support and equipment and providing the right kind of information (UN 2009: 7–8, 12 and 17). For these to make sense and to become embedded in practice social workers need to see them in action and that is what the interview excerpts with Aine will attempt to illustrate. In terms of what else social workers can practically do to get the best beginning, following some or all of the ideas outlined in Table 5.1 might help.

The focus of the beginnings stage is to ensure that the child knows who the social worker is, what their job is and what the purpose of the visit is. This information has to be shared in a clear and accessible manner (Koprowska 2008: 53; Trevithick 2005: 118–9; Wilson *et al.* 2008: 303; UN 2009: 26, para. 134; also, article 13 UNCRC). In order to ensure this and to be sure that this process reflects the individuality and the skills and abilities of each child it is important for the social worker to think about ways, other than verbal exchange, through which this information might be imparted (Trevithick 2005: 119; Marchant 2008: 151–8; UN 2009: 17, paras 80–3). Hence Table 5.1 illustrates that social workers might want to include the use of postcards, photos, small picture albums and other materials.

Table 5.1 also assumes that children will want to have a conversation with their social worker. However some children will not. In these cases this choice is to be respected (UN 2009: 6, para. 16). However, it is also important to be clear that the child's reluctance is not down to the social worker's failure to give appropriate, accessible, clear information in a suitable format or the social worker's failure to take account of a particular context that might act as a hindrance to a child engaging in a conversation

Table 5.1 Beginnings stage of the communication process

Beginnings	*What you can do to help*
Introduce yourself	Have a small photo album with a photo of you, you and your car, you outside your office, you with colleagues or you talking with children and families. Have a postcard with picture, name, number and job to leave with the child.
Give information about your job title and role	Check out whether the child knows what a social worker is and explain to them if they are not sure. You can say that a social worker is someone who tries to help children and families who have problems.
Confirm the reason for your visit	Check out whether the child knows why you are visiting. Explain the purpose (i.e. 'I got a telephone call from your teacher who is worried about you'). Seek the child's permission to enter into a conversation about this.
Set out the room together	Lay out and introduce the materials to be used in the interview and the reason you are using them. Give the child a choice about whether they wish to use them or not.
Construct initial conversation around non-threatening issues	Choose a topic that you know is either neutral or non-threatening (this could include the weather or your journey, for example).
Use skills to help the child feel at ease	Use skills of mirroring and pacing to develop rapport and to help a child feel at ease.

(UN 2009: 26, para. 134). As stated, social workers are required to respect the choices of young children while also making it clear that they will be available for them to talk with if they wish on another occasion.

Having outlined what helps make a good beginning to an interview there is now the opportunity to see these principles in practice in the following interview excerpt, which involves the introductory process with Aine.

EXERCISE

Take time to read the following excerpt involving the introduction to Aine, and answer the following questions:

- Find examples where I introduce myself, give information about job title and role, confirm reason for visit and seek permission to talk.
- Find where and how Aine and I engaged in the process of setting up the interview room in a way that Aine was happy with.
- List examples where you think things could have been done differently and/or better.

KW: Now Aine do you remember me asking you whether you could help me understand a little bit about your thoughts and feelings?

Aine: Yep.

KW: Yep?

Aine: [*Nods head to say yes.*]

KW: And would you like to do that today?

Aine: [*Nods*] Look! Are these baby things [*pointing to craft materials on the table that include a pack of stickers designed around the theme of a newborn baby*]?

KW: Yes.

Aine: These are baby things.

KW: Shall we take some of these out of their boxes and put them on the table in case we want to use them?

Aine: [*Nods.*]
        [*Gap in conversation where Aine and KW both set up the room and craft materials and sort the chairs out. Aine leads in terms of selecting the craft materials and placing chairs where she wants. She decides not to use chairs to sit at the low table but crouches at the table on her knees. KW copies.*]

KW: Can you remember [. . .] what my job is with you today?

Aine: No.

KW: Do you remember that little leaflet with the pictures on the front?

Aine: [*Nods.*]

KW: And it told you about some special work I am doing to find out what children like you think and feel?

Aine: Ah hah.

KW: And that my work is to help social workers do their job even better?

Aine: [*Nods.*]

KW: One of the things I do with children is these boxes [*KW shows Aine a shoebox*], where, on the outside, they make what they think they look like – right? And then on the inside is all the things that go on in your head

and your heart all your thoughts and feelings.
[*Aine begins to work on her box sticking down stickers. There is a pause in conversation while she does this. KW watches.*]

KW: Aine, do you remember talking about Ann and Angela [*referring to conversation about her sisters that had taken place on the way into the room*]?

Aine: There you can use the scissors for me. [KW *helps Aine cut out a piece of material.*]

From this excerpt it can be seen that I attempted to establish rapport with Aine and create the right conditions for our communication by clarifying my role, the purpose of our meeting and through the process of setting up the room for our time together. These principles reflect the child rights-based approach outlined in the previous chapter. In particular, in terms of addressing the power imbalance in the conversation, while it was me that controlled the process of arranging the actual interview, some control was given back to Aine in the interview process by seeking her agreement to continue the interview (rather than merely assuming that she will want to do this) and by her exercising choice as to the way the room was organized. More control could have been given by allowing Aine to choose freely from the materials on offer rather than me directing her to a particular method which, in this case, was the shoebox, a method which is discussed in more detail in Chapter Six.

EXERCISE
Think about conversations you have had with children and consider the following questions:

•   Think about what types of topic should you begin an interview with.
•   Think of a few examples and give reasons as to why you think they might be a good way of beginning.

Another important way of giving control to a child in a conversation is by initiating a discussion around an issue that you know they do not find threatening or intrusive. This aspect of the beginnings stage is illustrated below in a conversation that leads on from Aine and myself setting up the room and Aine talking about her sisters, Ann and Angela, as she walked into the room:

KW: Ah hah. And what were you telling me about Ann and Angela?
Aine: That they moved house.
KW: And have you seen them in their new house?
Aine: No haven't seen their new house.
KW: And you told me it might be sad when they move?
Aine: Yes.
KW: Why did it make you sad?
Aine: Because it wasn't fair.
KW: Because it wasn't fair?
Aine: Move house too.
KW: You wanted to move house too? So why did you want to move house?

Aine:	Cos I didn't like my other house there, right over [*referring to the box she is decorating*].
KW:	That's it. You didn't like your house that you are in and you wanted to go to a new house? [*Gap while Aine plays with craft materials.*] And why don't you like the house that you are in?
Aine:	Cos it's not good.
KW:	Cos it's not good? And which bits are not good about it?
Aine:	Cos I go on a naughty chair.
KW:	Oh. Cos you go on a naughty chair. Oh dear! And when do you come off the naughty chair?
Aine:	Don't know. I **DO NOT** know [*saying words in an exaggerated American accent!*].
KW:	So you don't like it cos there's a naughty chair?
Aine:	Yeah.
	[*Aine proceeds to look around and talk about the room we are in. She sees a mirror. Aine and KW chat about the height chart on the wall and then Aine returns to her drawing*].
KW:	So Aine who lives in the house that you're in?
Aine:	My daddy.
KW:	Your daddy and?
Aine:	Mummy and my brother and [*Aine does not finish sentence*] . . .
KW:	And?
Aine:	Me and [*Aine does not finish sentence. Voice trails off. Her thoughts seem to preoccupy her*] . . .
KW:	And?
Aine:	Doggy. I've got two doggies.
KW:	What's your doggies names?
Aine:	Boots and Dempster.
KW:	And how long have you lived with your mummy, your daddy and your dogs?
Aine:	29.
KW:	29. And where were you living before that?
Aine:	At my mummy's house, at my other mummy's house.

This excerpt shows that the topics introduced at the start of an interview are an important consideration to help put children at ease and reduce their possible feelings of anxiety or fear. As stated earlier it is best to start with a neutral issue or an issue that the child feels confident in exploring (Lefevre 2008: 133). In this part of the conversation with Aine this involved a discussion about her sisters. Although I took the lead in terms of introducing the topic it seemed a safe one to start with as she had already raised the issue. Again this action was important in signalling to Aine that she would have some control in the interview process. An indication that Aine felt comfortable with the beginning of our conversation together was that she quickly moved from identifying who was in her foster family to expressing some of her feelings about these matters. This reflected a combination of building rapport and creating the right conditions, particularly in terms of providing the right kind of information and materials and respecting her individuality. For example, it took time for Aine to choose and then set out the materials and the room and it was crucial that her pace was respected.

In the above conversations with Aine, although not completely apparent from the transcript, further important skills in rapport-building included mirroring and pacing. These involved copying the speech (volume, speed and tone of voice), language (the words used) and body language (hand movements, gestures, resting elbows on table, sitting with legs crossed) of Aine. Mirroring and pacing are subtle processes, often not carried out consciously, where people often replicate the signals and behaviour of the other. They convey a non-judgemental attitude and create feelings of safety and security for the child involved. It is probably this that leads people to feel they are 'clicking' with someone. Being aware of these skills helps reduce some of the power differential between the social worker and the child (Lefevre 2008: 130–45). It is especially important to be aware of the issue of power in relation to children because, as Koprowska (2008: 96) argues,

> [a]dults are inherently more powerful than children [and] vulnerable and disadvantaged children, especially younger ones, are highly susceptible to adult influence. They defer to adults, are sensitized to verbal and non-verbal cues and comply. We have to be careful not to cue them into telling us what they think we want to hear.

It is possible to find examples of verbal mirroring in these conversations with Aine. The use of the word 'doggies' for example and acceptance of Aine's description of the length of her placement in foster care as '29' are examples. These skills are reflective of a child rights-based approach in which the individuality, the choices and the contributions of Aine are respected, valued and encouraged (UN 2005; UN 2009: 26–7, para. 134).

Middle

The middle of the communication process represent a stage where the process and quality of information exchange and also the level of interaction should deepen (Wilson *et al.* 2008: 306). This stage of the communication process raises a number of important issues for social workers to consider, including: their skills base, recognizing and managing emotions (in themselves and the child), recognizing and respecting the social agency of the child (the child's own choices and contributions in the direction and content of the conversation) and the use of methods to facilitate the conversation. Each of these four issues will be illustrated through my own conversations with Aine.

Social worker's skills base

EXERCISE

- List what skills you think you might need to communicate with children in the middle stage of an interview/meeting/visit.
- Consider whether any of those skills you have listed are more important than the others?
- Reconsider your answers when you have read the next conversation with Aine.

The conversation below continues where the last one, noted earlier, left off. The purpose of my conversation with Aine was to explore a number of key questions with her – namely, What did she remember about home? Did she understand why she was removed from her parents' home and therefore the reasons why she was in care? What were her feelings? And did she have an opportunity to convey her perspectives to help inform decision-making about her? This is a long excerpt. However, and as explained earlier, this is important because these are Aine's words; they demonstrate quite clearly that she is able to convey information about difficult issues competently and that she has the capacity to engage in a sustained and lengthy conversation.

KW:	And who lived in your other mummy and daddy's [birth parents] house?
Aine:	[*Pause*] My mummy and my daddy and my brother Andrew and my two sisters.
KW:	Do you know why you don't live with your mummy, daddy, Andrew, Ann-Marie and Angela?
Aine:	Yep.
KW:	And why is that?
Aine:	Cos I was cheeky to them.
KW:	[*Later in interview*] And when you lived at your house in Old Way what, tell me what happened every day.
Aine:	Ann-Marie wanted to steal my toys and I wanted to steal her toys and then we started fighting.
KW:	So you and Ann-Marie started fighting a lot? And were the toys upstairs or downstairs?
Aine:	Upstairs.
KW:	And did you spend a lot of time in your bedrooms?
Aine:	Yeah cos I spent a lot of time staying in there playing and fighting and putting poo on our head.
KW:	You put poo on your head?
Aine:	Yeah where it comes out your bum.
KW:	[*Later in the interview*] So the poo that comes out your bum you get out your bum and you just put it on there [*pointing to head*]?
Aine:	And then we put it all over our walls.
KW:	Did you? And why did you do that?
Aine:	Cos it comes on our nappies and we took our nappies off.
KW:	I see, so the poo comes out of your bum into your nappies, you took your nappies off?
Aine:	And I had a nappy.
KW:	And you had a nappy? So you took your nappy off, got poo and put it there [*pointing to head and walls*] and then who sorted that out for you?
Aine:	No one.
KW:	No one sorted it out. Did anyone clean your hair?
Aine:	Dad and Ann-Marie screamed.
KW:	[*Later in interview*] And how did it make you feel when you were putting poo from your nappies on your head and on the walls?
Aine:	Not good.
KW:	Not good. No.
KW:	[*Later in interview*] What else went on when you were at home?

Aine:	Don't know and then I would throw my mattress off my bed and jumped around on it.
KW:	Did you ever play anything else in your bedrooms?
Aine:	No.
KW:	And then what happened when you were not in your bedrooms?
Aine:	Not nowhere.
KW:	Did you used to go downstairs at all?
Aine:	I had a lock.
KW:	You had a lock and where was the lock?
Aine:	On the top.
KW:	On the top. Whereabouts on the top?
Aine:	On the door.
KW:	[*Later in interview*] So who used to put the lock on your door? You know when you went in through your door? Who put the lock on?
Aine:	No one. My daddy did when I went to bed.
KW:	Why do you think he did this Aine?
Aine:	Cos he kept thinking in case I get out.
KW:	Did you used to try and get out then?
Aine:	No.

Of course probably the first thing that is striking is how appalling Aine's experiences were and how she is able to convey them so lucidly. It is very difficult to imagine a child of Aine's age being locked in her room and neglected to the extent where she regularly smeared faeces on her head and on the walls. Her memories are likely to evoke strong emotional responses from those who listen to her account.

EXERCISE
Before continuing, write a list of your emotional responses, keep them to one side and we will return to them shortly to engage in proper exercises and a full discussion.

The first issue to be considered in relation to the middle stage of communication is the social workers' skills base. Table 5.2 provides a summary of the *listening skills, questioning skills and responding skills* that are used to successfully navigate the way through the middle stage of the interview. For those interested, each of these is described in detail elsewhere (Koprowska 2008: 82–9; Trevithick 2005: 140–89).

Some may mistakenly interpret Table 5.2 as implying that during the course of an interview these skills are exercised by social workers in an ordered, hierarchical fashion. This is not the case. All three interweave throughout the course of a conversation with some more prominent at certain points than others.

In relation to my own *listening skills* in the conversation with Aine, sometimes I listened with silence (Wilson *et al.* 2008: 310–11) and sometimes I responded to Aine's comment with a comment or a question. What is important, but cannot be well reflected in written excerpts, is an attitude of listening with non-verbal responses such as head nods, positioning (leaning body forward or with head to one side, for example) and facial/eye movements (Koprowska 2008: 38; Trevithick 2005: 119–21). These cues

Table 5.2 Communication skills base with children

Skill	Skill in action
Listening skills	Listening is an active rather than passive activity. It involves being attentive, concentrating, responding and searching for meaning. It means showing interest, empathy and support. Finally, it involves using silence where appropriate.
Questioning skills	The use of open, closed and probing questions.
Responding skills	The use of verbal skills in reflecting, paraphrasing, clarifying and summarizing.

are very important in conveying the message to the child that they are being listened to attentively and completely.

Good use of *questioning skills* is also central to any interview process, with the aim of the interviewer being to uncover facts, feelings, reasons and detail. There are four types of questioning: open, closed, probing and leading (Trevithick 2005: 140–89). An open question is usually prefixed with 'how', 'why' or 'what' and is designed to allow the interviewee to reveal information with them taking the lead. An example of an open question in the interview with Aine is:

KW: And when you lived at your house in Old Way what, tell me what happened every day.

A closed question results in a short response rather than detailed elaboration. Often a closed question is designed to gather specific information about a particular issue. Examples of closed questions from the interview with Aine include:

KW: Did you used to go downstairs at all?
KW: You had a lock and where was the lock?
KW: On the top. Whereabouts on the top?

The above might also be counted as a series of small probing questions where I was gathering detail on a sensitive issue, in this case Aine's experience of being locked in her bedroom. A probing question can be open or closed and is used to begin to touch upon an area of interest but often indirectly. Probing questions can rely on a child's recall ('Tell me about what you did in the morning') or they can rely on recognition ('Was the lock metal or wooden?'). Generally it is felt that questions that rely on young children's recall help children explore and express their experiences more freely (Larsson and Lamb 2009). The last type of questions are leading questions, so called because they are suggestive to children. Examples include 'you did come downstairs sometimes didn't you?' or 'you must have felt very angry mustn't you?' Because they can be experienced as coercive and constraining they are best avoided.

As Aine started to reveal her memories she required reassurance from me that what she said had been listened to. Good *responding skills* include the following: reflecting (i.e. I hear and understand your feelings), paraphrasing (i.e. I hear and understand the content of what you are saying), summarizing (i.e. similar to paraphrasing but usually with longer summaries) and clarifying (confirming the accuracy of what has been said and sorting out confusions) (Trevithick 2005: 164–9). These should occur in a context in which the child feels that they are valued, respected and accepted (UN 1989, 2005, 2009). Examples of these skills can be seen in the following excerpt:

KW: And did you spend a lot of time in your bedrooms?

Aine: Yeah cos I spent a lot of time staying in there playing and fighting and putting poo on our head.

KW: You put poo on your head [*reflecting*]?

Aine: Yeah where it comes out your bum.

KW: [. . .] So the poo that comes out your bum you get out your bum and you just put it on there [*pointing to head*] [*paraphrasing*]?

Recognizing and managing emotions

EXERCISE
Return to the list of emotional responses that you made earlier and consider the following:

- What were your emotional responses?
- What might have been Aine's emotional responses in the circumstances she describes?
- Why is it important to be emotionally self-aware?
- What strategies can you think of to help you manage your own emotions?
- What strategies can you think of to help you manage Aine's emotions and also to help her manage her own emotions?
- What were your other reactions? And how might these be dealt with?

As stated earlier, it is likely that reading about Aine's memories of her home life will have evoked strong emotional responses. If social workers accept that young children can share their views, and if social workers have built a rapport and established the right conditions for the interview, we must be prepared to listen to what children might then go on to tell us. It is not easy to listen to Aine's memories. Her interview stirs up all sorts of emotional responses towards the parents including horror ('how could they do this?'), anger ('how dare they do this!') through to confusion ('why did they do this?'). There are also emotional responses towards Aine including sadness, anger and/ or shock ('your experiences were appalling'), sorrow and guilt ('so sorry that no one helped you earlier') through to admiration ('I am amazed at your resilience').

How was it possible for Aine to describe her own feelings and how was it possible for me to manage Aine's emotions (interpersonal skills) and my own (intrapersonal skills)? Morrison (2007) and Howe (2008) state that these interpersonal and intrapersonal skills comprise what is termed emotional intelligence. First, in relation to *my own emotions*, emotional intelligence is crucial to building meaningful relationships and communicating with young children. It enables children to feel safe, to express difficult feelings without fear of rejection or judgement and to begin the process of making sense of the past, the present and what might be in the future. As highlighted through the interviews with social workers in Chapter Three, those who avoid confronting and dealing with their own emotions and/or the emotions of children are more likely to have distant relationships with them which can, in turn, and as demonstrated so vividly in the child abuse inquiries, contribute to practice in which children's safety and well-being are compromised. As Morrison argues,

> [a] lack of self-awareness or suppression of emotion may result in important information being missed, either about the presence of external dangers or about intrusions from the worker's own experience, which may distort observation and assessment.
>
> (Morrison 2007: 255)

Morrison (2007) and Howe (2008) discuss how being emotionally intelligent involves a process of understanding and recognizing, labelling and expressing, and managing and controlling emotions. How does this work in practice? In relation to my emotions, while I attempted to keep them visibly in check during the interview with Aine, I did nonetheless experience emotional responses. I remember being shocked almost to the point of disbelief ('Did I hear Aine right?' 'Did she just say that she had put poo over her head?'), appalled ('The smell from which there could have been no escape') and guilty on behalf of the profession as a whole ('How could we, as social workers, have allowed things to get so bad?'). The key though was not to express these emotions during the course of the interview because this could convey the impression that I was either not coping, did not believe and/or could not listen. Having said this, rather than burying these emotional responses completely I later had space with the supervisor of my research to explore these feelings and my own management of them.

Second, in relation to *Aine's emotions*, the interview process allowed her to explore, express and vent her emotions safely without her feeling that they were being judged, curtailed, minimized or dismissed. An example of this is where, during the course of the interview, Aine expressed her feelings of sadness as follows:

KW: And what was messy about Andrew's room? What kinds of things were messy in his room?

Aine: [*Delay in response and silent play*] All his play stations and his pens an all and his bed was all messy.

KW: Was it?

Aine: [*Lets out a half-scream*]

KW: And what was messy in his bed?

Aine: All of his bedware, clothes off and his sheets were minging [meaning filthy and/or dirty] and he was moaning.

KW: And what was he moaning about?

Aine: Cos he didn't get to eat anything and he got too much bed.

KW: And so he didn't get to [*interrupted by Aine letting out a loud and unpleasant baby Waaaah noise*]. Oh is that what he used to do?

Aine: Yes.

KW: Is that the noise he used to make?

Aine: Yeah.

KW: I see and how did you feel when he made that noise?

Aine: Sad.

KW: Sad. Yes. [. . .] What do you do when you're sad?

Aine: [*No response.*]
            [*Aine engages in silent play. KW watches Aine smearing paint all over her paper in circular motions.*]

Aine engaged in the action of smearing paint all over the paper in circular motions with both hands for several minutes. When she was asked what her actions reminded her of, she responded:

KW: When you are doing this does it remind you of anything?
Aine: Um um.
KW: What does it remind you of?
Aine: Not to scream in my house.
KW: Not to scream. And what happens if you scream?
Aine: You get a sore throat.
KW: What else does that remind you of? [*Silence in interview as KW watches Aine moving hands in a circular motion across paper.*] Does it remind you of anything?
Aine: No. [*Delay. More silent play.*] And Ann-Marie did put stuff [poo] in her own gob.
KW: Did she?
Aine: Yep and I didn't get to do stuff. Write things.
KW: Write things down?

The important point about these excerpts is that Aine expressed her emotions vividly. Her mimicry of her brother's screams was loud and piercing. Her actions of smearing paint on paper were a vivid re-enactment of the smearing that went on in the bedroom. While both were shocking, and could easily have led to attempts by me to cut their expression short, the process of managing Aine's emotions involved supporting her to make sense of them. Hence, in the conversation, when I asked her what the smearing actions reminded her of she said they reminded her not to scream. They also reminded her that she saw her sister put faeces in her mouth.

   Third, in relation to the management of the process more generally, the use of empathy was a key skill which Trevithick describes as 'trying to understand, as carefully and sensitively as possible, the nature of another person's experience, their own unique point of view and what meaning that carries for the individual [in this case Aine]' (Trevithick 2005: 153–4). She was not interrupted by me in this process but supported until she brought this aspect of the conversation to an end and it moved on to another issue. Similar processes were at play when Aine explored, later in the interview, her feelings about her removal from the family home.

KW: Who brought you over to your new mummy and daddy? How did you get there?
Aine: A girl brung me.
KW: And were you happy to be there?
Aine: No sad. I went to my granny's house over and across the road near to my mummy's and then I came there [meaning foster placement]. I went there.
KW: And did you understand why you couldn't live at home anymore?
Aine: No!

KW:	Did no one sit down and tell you?
Aine:	No.
KW:	Do you think they should have done?
Aine:	What?
KW:	Told you why you couldn't live at home?
Aine:	[*No answer.*]
KW:	So this lady just brought you over to there and you didn't know why?
Aine:	Yeah.
KW:	Goodness me.
Aine:	So that was not fair.
KW:	So that was not fair? And what would have been fair Aine?
Aine:	That I would get to see my mummy and I didn't want to move and then they left me.
KW:	And that wasn't fair?
Aine:	No.

Aine's emotional responses to her removal are probably quite surprising in that one might have expected Aine to be relieved, grateful and/or happy at having been removed from such appalling conditions. However, she expressed none of the expected emotions. She felt angry, let down and abandoned. The process of managing her feelings included me acknowledging and accepting them rather than admonishing them. Skills such as reflecting back, paraphrasing and summarizing were crucial to this.

Recognizing and respecting children's social agency

So far it has been seen that a successful interview depends on developing a good rapport, the use of good listening, questioning and responding skills, sensitivity to non-verbal skills and the ability to recognize and manage emotions. A further crucial component to the success of the middle stage is social workers' ability to respect, accept and value the social agency of the child.

EXERCISE
Think of young children that you know either professionally or personally and consider the following questions:

- What do you understand by the term 'social agency'?
- How might children show agency in the course of a conversation?
- Why is it important to recognize and respect children's agency?

In the examples below I provide illustrations of Aine's strategies to exercise control over the pace, depth and direction of the interview. These included Aine's use of silences, distraction and deflection, humour, boundary-testing and re-enactment of past behaviours. These are types of social agency through which Aine challenged, controlled and took charge of the direction and dynamics within the conversation. Aine's responses should be a reminder to social workers that Aine is a person with her own personality and perspectives who is to be valued, respected and treated with dignity (UN 2009). In this case this means respecting the choices and control that she exerts, while simultaneously seeking meaning and understanding about these. It is this aspect of communicating with young children that is often missing in books and training materials. And yet it is this aspect of communication (i.e. what children say and do themselves) that is so important in terms of respecting, protecting and fulfilling young children's rights and in further challenging our own limited view of young children's social competence (Alderson 2000/2008). The remainder of the chapter considers each type of social agency – namely, use of silences; distraction and deflection, humour, boundary-testing and re-enactment of past behaviours in turn.

At certain points in the interview excerpts included in this chapter, Aine found her memories difficult to talk about. It was not that she did not want to talk about them but just that she found them emotionally challenging. As we have seen, she used *silences* to regain her composure and gather her thoughts before moving on to discuss her memories. The challenge to me as the interviewer was to not retreat from the poignancy of these moments and/or to try and rescue Aine from the pain of her own feelings by denying her an opportunity to express them. We both had to 'stay with the silences' (Koprowska 2008; Wilson *et al.* 2008: 310–11). Trevithick (2005: 175) explains this process further when she states that 'the assumption is that talking is better than not talking and that nothing is being communicated when silence prevails. This is not the case, because words can be used to create or kill real dialogue, to conceal rather than to reveal'. These processes are illustrated in the interview excerpts above where Aine was talking about her lack of food, her brother's room and his distress, and her sister Ann-Marie putting faeces in her own mouth.

When Aine started describing some of her experiences of loss – namely, of her granny and pet dog – associated with her move into care she used *distraction and deflection* to reduce the intensity of the interview and to retain control over her own emotions. By turning her attention, thoughts and effort to the craftwork she was able to create 'thinking space' to recover and compose herself sufficiently before proceeding with the interview. This can be seen in the following:

KW: And you said to me that your granny lived nearby did she?
Aine: [*Pause from Aine.*]
KW: Did she live next door?
Aine: [*Aine does not answer question*] Oh it's the wrong way [*referring to piece of craft work she is making*].
         [*Aine and KW talk about the craft materials, cutting and who is going to do it. Aine seems pre-occupied.*]
KW: And who else lives in Allwood that you know?
         [*Aine deflects from answering by making comments on her craftwork. Looks to KW for next question.*]
KW: Aine, who else lives in Allwood?
Aine: DOGGY [*shouting this word out*].
KW: What was your doggy's name?
Aine: ANGUS [*proceeds to laugh out loud with forced laughter*].
         [*Aine is upset at having to leave granny and the dog behind when she came into care. Aine and KW return to the discussion about Aine's craftwork.*]

As noted in the earlier discussion she used humour, in this case the use of a theatrical American accent, to manage her exasperation at her foster carers' practice of using the naughty chair. The use of this accent brought smiles and laughter from both Aine and I, which performed the function of diffusing Aine's feelings of frustration and anger. The diffusion did not detract from the content of what was said, the seriousness of what was said or the strength with which the opinion was held. Rather, it allowed Aine to create a space for herself to keep her feelings in check.

Similarly, in one of the other conversations where she talked about Andrew screaming, she gave an example of how his screaming sounded to her. The screaming was loud, painful and quite shocking. It felt as if Aine was trying to induce in me the feelings that she had experienced when she heard Andrew's screaming, including feelings of panic, shock and embarrassment and as a way of *testing boundaries*. I felt that this was, in part, a test of my authority (what was I going to do about it and what could I do about it?). This process was managed by not 'giving in' to Aine's testing but by seeking clarification from her and acknowledging her strength of feeling.

As already noted Aine *re-enacted some past behaviours* (smearing actions through the use of paint and paper) when discussing some of her feelings. As she told me her story I felt as if we had been locked in the room together and that I was observing what she did in that room to cope. My role in these parts of the conversation where Aine was demonstrating different types of social agency was just that, an observer, passing no judgement and not interfering with the process.

From the above section on children's social agency it can be seen that, far from young children being passive recipients of communication from adults, they use every opportunity to be active and to engage in reciprocal exchanges. It can be seen from the examples included that the term social agency refers to the capacity of children to exercise their own choices and control, and to change the dynamics, direction and decisions within their particular context. In communicating with young children social workers need to be clear that while it is they who set up the interview, with an agenda often controlled by them, it is possible for young children, within the constraints of the interview context, to operate their own choices, control and changes. These exchanges may be verbal and/or non-verbal.

Social workers need to have flexibility, insight and wisdom to tune in to and respond to the choices and controls that children exert. As McLeod (2007) notes in her own research with older children in care, it is important to respect the choices and controls that children are exerting, particularly in situations where they feel they have had little previous control in communication processes. This might involve practical tasks such as children choosing what it is that they wish to talk about and how they wish to do this. This child rights-based approach respects and values the contributions of children to the communication process. In this sense the communication process is based on reciprocity where there is an exchange of ideas, control of the process is shared rather than dominated by the social worker and ideas that emerge are the result of children and their social workers working in collaboration. These processes also draw attention to the importance of understanding communication in its broadest sense and of according, for example, as much weight to body language during an interview encounter as to the spoken word (Connolly 2008; Christensen and James, 2008b).

Methods to facilitate the communication process

So far, this chapter has considered the following as crucial to the process of social workers' communication: skills base, ability to recognize and manage emotions (in themselves and the child) and ability to recognize and respect the social agency of the child (the child's own choices and contributions to the direction and content of the conversation). One last area that will be touched on this chapter and developed further in the next concerns social workers' use of methods to facilitate conversations with young children.

As seen in earlier conversations with Aine, she used paint and craftwork during her conversations with me. In one of my early conversations with Aine I outlined to her the use of shoeboxes to depict feelings. Aine engaged with this particular method immediately to explore her views about herself and her feelings. During the course of the interview she constructed shoeboxes depicting herself and her feelings. On her first box she constructed an image of herself on the outside of the box to illustrate what she looked like and wanted to look like to others around her. The comparison between her description of herself at home (hair and head covered in faeces, naked and physically constrained for lengthy periods in one room) was a stark comparison with the image she constructed of herself in which she was neat, clean, sparkly and a dancer.

In the inside of her first box, shown in Figure 5.1, she depicted her inner feelings – the ones that people do not see – that focused on her dogs, smearing and her foster carers' back garden. The paper with sparkles on it was initially smeared with paint and then at a later stage sprinkled with glitter to represent the garden of her new foster home. Alongside this, Figure 5.2 shows the outside of Aine's second box, which captures her interests and hobbies.

She said that she liked cycling, dancing and animals (pink feather). On the inside of the second box Aine made a smaller box. Inside the smaller box she placed pieces of

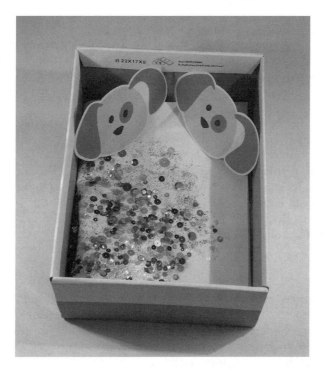

Figure 5.1 The inside of Aine's first reality box.

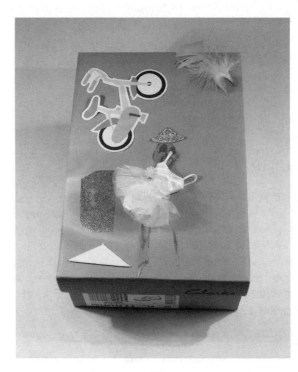

Figure 5.2 The outside of Aine's second reality box.

paper with feelings on them folded over and covered by a lid as shown in Figures 5.3 and 5.4. To read the feelings the lid has to be removed. Reflecting the personal nature of its contents, it was important to seek Aine's permission to take out the contents of the little box to photograph them even though she had asked me to write the labels on her behalf.

The feelings in her box represented the friends that were important to her and also her longing to remain connected with her mother and father. The craftwork with Aine was particularly important because it enabled Aine and I to establish a good rapport. Furthermore, the methods provided a vehicle through which she and I could explore her thoughts and feelings. Importantly, during this Aine used the methods to control the depth, pace and content of the interview. Lastly, the methods served as a visual representing the depth of Aine's feelings and experiences. These and other issues related to participatory methods are explored in the next chapter.

Endings

Ending conversations with young children is as important as beginning them as well (Trevithick 2005: 181–7; Wilson *et al.* 2008: 306–7). In my research there are several examples of young children who, once they had engaged in the interview, did not want it to end. In the following excerpt there are some practical ideas about how to end communication with young children well:

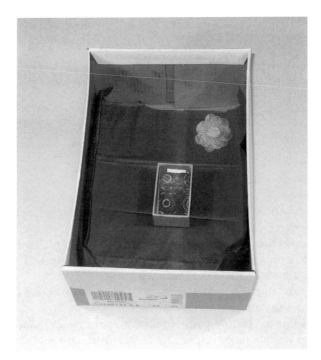

Figure 5.3 The inside of Aine's second reality box.

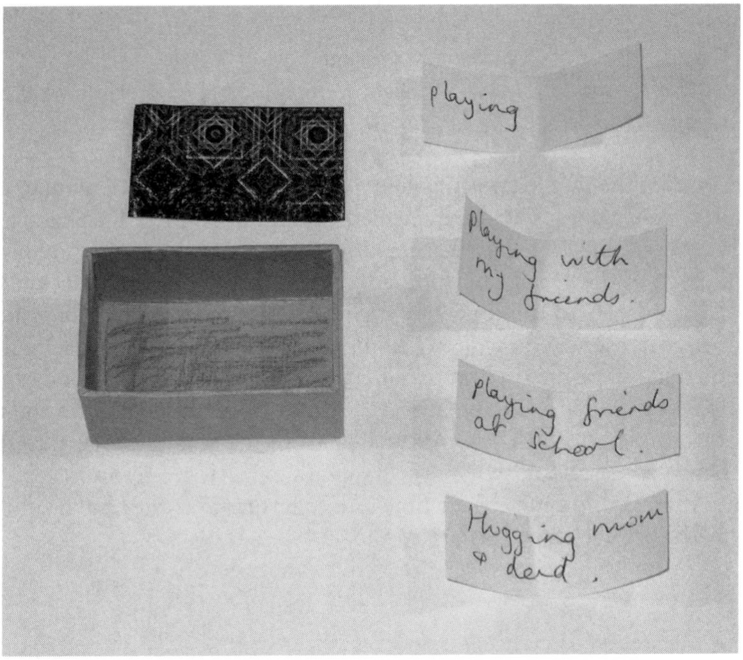

Figure 5.4 The contents of Aine's second reality box.

EXERCISE

Consider the following and make notes of your answers:

- Why is it important to end conversations well?
- What are some of the common mistakes made in ending communication with each other?
- What types of strategy could you use to end a conversation with a young child well?

KW: Aine can you see the clock?

Aine: [*Nods head.*]

KW: It is nearly time for us to finish. Shall we tidy up together?

Aine: [*No answer.*]

            [*Aine continues to play. KW lets Aine continue to play for a few minutes.*]

KW: Aine it is time for us to finish. Let's tidy up together. If you like you can choose a pack of stickers to take with you.

Aine: Can I take these [*pointing to pack of stickers*] and one of those [*holding pom-pom in hand*]?

KW: Sure. Is this the picture you are taking to your foster-mum? Let's put it over there so we don't lose it [*packing away*]. You have told me lots about your memories and feelings today.

Aine: Ah-ha.

KW: I think it might be a good idea for you to spend some more time doing this. What do you think?

Aine: Ah-ha.

KW: OK. I will talk to your social worker.

            [*KW and Aine discuss again items being made for foster-mum and interview terminated. Process of clearing up takes several minutes.*]

It is important that the interview is finished in a timely and sensitive manner so that the child is not left feeling confused, used, rejected and/or abandoned. Endings are therefore a process that should be anticipated and planned for. To begin the ending process, and if there is a clock in the room, the ending can be indicated by showing the child that when the big hand gets to number 9 (for example) this means that the time together needs to finish. Another useful way to begin the ending process is by packing materials away. I found that where children were reluctant to begin this process of disengagement they could be encouraged by being allowed to take an item away with them (such as stickers, for example). It is also important, as part of the ending process, to summarize the main issues discussed and what will happen next. Most importantly, it is always important to thank children for their time and to ensure that they have your details to take away with them. These ideas are summarized in Table 5.3.

Summary

Through the use of a detailed case study this chapter has outlined the key stages of the interview, the processes involved and the issues that emerge in each stage and how

Table 5.3 Endings stage of the communication process

Endings	What you can do to help
Warning	Five minutes before the end of the interview let the child know that the interview will shortly be coming to an end.
Summing up	Involve the child in summing up the main issues that have been discussed today.
Clearing away	Begin to clear up the room together.
Thanking	Thank the child for their time and for their input. Let the child know that you have valued your conversation together.
Planning ahead	Explain what will happen next. Ensure the child has your contact details on a postcard.

these should be managed. The chapter has shown that communication with young children involves establishing rapport, creating the right conditions, the confident use of listening, questioning and responding skills, appropriate management of feelings and emotions, respect for the choices of the child and the use of methods to facilitate the interview process. Most importantly, the chapter has shown how all of these processes and practices are reflective of and grounded in a child rights-based approach. The next chapter considers the use of methods in more detail, drawing upon examples from other case studies from my research.

6 Communicating with young children
Methods

Summary of chapter content

This chapter outlines some of the key participatory methods that can be used to communicate with young children. It begins with an overview of the key issues that need to be considered by social workers in using these methods before outlining each of the main methods in turn. An exercise at the end of the chapter will help social workers think about how these might apply to their daily practice.

Introduction

As has been made clear through previous chapters, developing relationships and communication is crucial to safeguarding children and, moreover, it is not an option but is required practice. Childcare legislation and related policy makes it clear that social workers must seek, listen to and take seriously the views of children on all matters concerning them. Furthermore, research reviews of participatory methods illustrate the broad range of methods available for work with children (Clark and Statham 2005; O'Kane 2008). These range from digital methods such as flip cameras (to make podcasts) through to disposable cameras and the use of games, toys, stories, poems, construction and arts and crafts (Punch 2002a, 2002b; Darbyshire *et al.* 2005; Cook and Hess 2007). With regard to young children specifically a broad range of methods has been used to gain their views and perspectives (Clark and Moss 2001; Fasoli 2003; MacNaughton 2003; Clark and Statham 2005; Dockett and Perry 2007; Flewitt 2005; Winter 2010). Moreover, and as argued in this book and elsewhere, these methods can also be used by social workers to build relationships and communicate with young children (Hill 1997; Lefevre 2008; McLeod 2008b).

Indeed, many of these methods, as Hill (1997) and Lefevre (2008) note, have been an integral part of therapeutic social work practice for a long time. The benefits of communicating with young children have been illustrated in the previous chapter through the case study involving Aine. However, recent research with newly qualified social workers suggests that they often feel that they do not have the training or the methods to undertake this work with young children (CDWC Research Team 2009 unpublished). In particular, there is a lack of practical guidance about what methods to use and how exactly they should be employed. Moreover, there is a tendency to assume that the methods that are available are expensive and inaccessible.

This chapter take the view that it does not have to be this way. The purpose of this chapter is twofold: to show that the methods available are not necessarily expensive or elusive; and to show that it is not necessarily the methods as such that help communication but rather the way the child appropriates and uses them, together with the ways in which the social worker responds during the process of communication. The chapter begins by outlining the principles that should underpin the use of methods with young children before considering some of the types of method available. In each case, examples will be used to illustrate the points made. This, in turn, provides the basis from which, in the next chapter, in-depth case studies are used to demonstrate the holistic use of a variety of methods.

A child rights-based approach to the use of participatory methods

Previous chapters have focused on frameworks that emphasize the social agency of children and their rights and these two overarching themes should underpin the use of participatory methods in communicating with young children. In practice this means responding to the following six issues before, during and after the communication process: ethical issues, the choices and freedoms of children, the individuality of each child, the expressed views of the child, the power imbalances in the social worker–child relationship and the boundaries in that relationship (Barker and Weller 2003; Dockett and Perry 2007; Christensen and James 2008a; Connolly 2008). Each of these issues will now be considered in turn.

Ethical issues

From the case study of Aine in the last chapter it is clear that attention to ethical issues is paramount. Before the conversation begins children should be informed about the purpose of the conversation, the issues that are likely to be discussed and what will happen to the information they choose to share. Attention to these issues is reflective of a child rights-based approach. As stated in a recent UN report, General Comment No. 12 (UN 2009), and as noted in Chapter Four, a fundamental principle that should underpin all processes in which children are involved or asked to participate is that the processes are

> transparent and informative. Children must be provided with full, accessible, diversity-sensitive and age-appropriate information about their right to express their views freely and their views to be given due weight, and how this participation will take place, its scope, purpose and potential impact.
>
> (UN 2009: 26, para. (a))

Most notably, and in line with their legal responsibilities under childcare legislation, a social worker needs to make it clear to the child from the outset that if they talk about harm and danger they have experienced (or are experiencing) then this will have to be looked into further. It should also be made clear that their parents/ main carers and other professionals can receive a summary of the main issues discussed, as is also reflected in the requirement under childcare legislation to keep parents/carers informed of developments in relation to the child. Emotional support for the children, post-conversation if it is required, should also have been planned prior to the meeting with the child. This can involve having a person in a caring or therapeutic capacity, who knows the child well, being on hand to support the child.

During the conversation the social worker needs to be tuned in to the child's changing views about having the conversation. It may be that, at a certain point, the child wants the conversation to end or the subject matter to change or even just for the pace to alter. They may communicate this through their body language rather than words. Signs to look out for include looking away, fidgeting, walking around, focusing their attention on something else other than the conversation. The following chapter, which concerns itself with the application of skills and methods in real-life case examples, provides examples of young children's reactions and how these were responded to.

At the end of a conversation with a child there are further ethical issues to be addressed. For example, the decision about whether to use emotional support for the child should, where possible, be made in conjunction with the child. It could involve agreeing with the child that the social worker will contact them the next day and that if they still feel really upset the person identified to offer them support will be called upon. Where no issues of harm have been discussed, but where young children have revealed their views, they should be involved with the social worker in planning how, when, and in what format those views are shared with other professionals.

In the current research young children were given a choice as to what they wished to happen with their work: did they want to keep it themselves, or for me to look after it; and were they happy for it to be used, in photographs or 'real life', to help other social workers learn how to have better conversations with other young children. Children had a range of different responses. Some wanted to take their work and give it to their carers (but were happy for me to photograph it), one child did not want me to photograph their work and others wanted me to keep the work, photograph it and use it to help other social workers. In the current research the preservation of young children's anonymity was crucial. In social work practice while this may not necessarily be a consideration it is nonetheless important to treat children's work with respect and to involve them as fully as possible in the process of sharing their work with others. For example, in my job as a Guardian ad Litem I was involved in cases where the children's work, along with their words, was presented to the judges involved as a visual representation of their own wishes and feelings (as opposed to a descriptive summary provided by me). In other cases some judges saw the child, along with their work, so that the child could explain their perspective. Attention to these ethical issues is reflective of the respect for the individual worth and dignity of each individual child, which forms the basis of a child rights-based approach as noted in the UNCRC (UN 1989).

Respecting the choices and freedoms of young children

It may feel tokenistic to speak of respecting the choices and freedoms of the child when these seem to conflict with the constraints imposed by necessary child protection procedures. However, there are important ways in which the choices and freedoms of young children can still be respected. The most significant of these is the need to avoid making assumptions that young children will want to talk or what their preferred ways for communicating are.

There will be times, for example, when a child wants to just close down the conversation on a particular issue. As noted earlier young children may react to questions through shaking their heads, looking away, making noises or by moving around the room. Responses need to be tuned in to and respectful of these reactions rather than ignoring them. This is reflective of a child rights-based approach. The recent UN report notes that 'the child, however, has the right not to exercise this right. Expressing views is a choice for the child, not an obligation' (UN 2009: 6, para. 16). Similarly, a social worker may have brought a range of arts-based materials with them but the child then chooses not to use these but instead use objects in the room through which to express their feelings. In the current research children talked with me using telephones, computers and other props that were available in the room. Again, reflective of a child rights-based approach, responses need to be supportive and facilitative rather than judgemental and prescriptive.

What these examples illustrate is the fact that social workers need to accept that, with or without recourse to the particular methods on offer, some children will enjoy talking more than others and want to be more involved than others. Moreover, some will rely more on action and body language rather than the spoken word to express their views and some children will only want to talk for a short time and others will not want the communication to end (Butler and Williamson 1994; Backett-Milburn and McKie 1999; Christensen and James 2008b). Similarly, as noted by way of the examples in the preceding section, children may choose to do one of a number of things in relation to their completed work.

Supporting children in these choices and freedoms is crucial. However, having said this, in some instances it may just not be possible to follow through on respecting the choices of young children. An example of this occurred in relation to Aine who provided the focus for the last chapter. In talking with her, she expressed the wish that it would be better if her name accompanied her craftwork, as people would then know that it was her talking. However, her preference could not be honoured because the ethical requirement of anonymity overrode this. Also she did not want our conversation to end and this preference also could not be honoured as the room we were in was later booked for a supervised contact session involving another family.

The key point in all of this is to be upfront and open with the children about what is possible and what is not and, in cases where it is not possible to do as they request, to explain clearly why. Attention to children's choices and freedoms is an important aspect to children's participation rights, which include the right to express a view freely, (article 12 UNCRC, UN 1989) and the 'right to freedom of expression which includes freedom to seek, receive and impart information and ideas of all kinds, regardless of frontiers, either orally, in writing or in print, in the form of art, or through any other media of the child's choice' (article 13 UNCRC, UN 1989). Furthermore, attention to protection rights, as in the example of Aine above where her anonymity had to be protected, is an equally important aspect to a child rights-based approach where, as outlined in UN report General Comment No. 12 (UN 2009) and discussed in Chapter Four, the involvement of children has to be 'safe and sensitive to risk'. It goes on to state that

> [a]dults have a responsibility towards the children with whom they work and must take every precaution to minimize the risk to children of violence, exploitation or any other negative consequence of their participation. Action necessary to provide appropriate protection will include the development of a clear child-protection strategy, which recognizes the particular risks faced by some groups of children.
>
> (UN 2009: 27, para. (h))

Respecting the individuality of young children

With regard to respecting the individuality of young children, account needs to be taken of major group differences such as class, age, gender, disability, ethnicity or culture as well as the personality, temperament and likes/dislikes of each child. These principles are an inherent aspect to a child rights-based approach and adhered to in research (Punch 2002a, 2002b). For example, in my own work I met a young girl from Thailand who spoke good English but in our first meeting we found it difficult to establish a rapport even though she was keen on the arts-based methods made available. For our next meeting I included photographs from Thailand that I had gathered from my own travels. The inclusion of these photographs opened up the door to a vivid conversation about how she missed playing with her friends in her home village, running and cycling up and down the dirt tracks that surrounded the village and how she missed hearing the rain on the corrugated iron roof of her grandparents' home. What I attempted to do in this particular example was to demonstrate my respect for the individuality of this young child; in this case her Thai background. The same basic principles can be applied to other groups of children, including those with disabilities, for example, an issue which is further explored below in relation to power imbalances in the child–adult relationship (Marchant 2008).

Respecting children's views and feelings

Respect for children's views and valuing them means having a genuine interest in what the child shares, responding positively to the ways in which they choose to share their views (rather than judging, diverting or interfering in these processes), thanking them for their contributions and giving them feedback about how their views were considered in decisions and/or what influence they had. The final point is particularly important, and emphasized recently in a UN report, General Comment No. 12, which, as noted in Chapter Four, concerns itself with a child's right to be heard (UN 2009). It says that children's involvement has to be underpinned by accountability and this involves action whereby,

> in any research or consultative process, children must be informed as to how their views have been interpreted and used and, where necessary, provided with the opportunity to challenge and influence the analysis of the findings. Children are also entitled to be provided with clear feedback on how their participation has influenced any outcomes.

> (UN 2009: 27, para. (i))

In my work as a Guardian ad Litem, for example, I found the practice of one particular high court judge reflective of the great respect they placed on children's views when they wrote a letter to a child to explain that they had listened to their views and how and in what ways these had been taken into account in decision-making. The same judge also took time to explain why they had not been able to honour all of the child's wishes. Where possible the same principles have underpinned the current research although the ongoing involvement of the children in the dissemination of the findings has not been possible because that was not agreed as part of the ethical framework.

Attention to power imbalances

Another issue that social workers need to take into account in their conversations with young children is attention to power imbalances and how these differences might be addressed. Power imbalances obviously centre on the adult social worker–child relationship. On one level these power imbalances are impossible to overcome as, for example, social workers cannot reverse their professional and/or adult status. However, within a children's rights framework, there is a moral and ethical duty to acknowledge and work with the influences of these power relationships because otherwise they can lead to children's rights being ignored (Alderson 2000/2008; Danby and Farrell 2004; McLeod 2008b: 115–21).

The power imbalances, in relation to the adult–child relationship, as indicated in earlier chapters, are structured around all sorts of assumptions, made by adults and children alike, regarding differential levels of competence, experience, wisdom and insight that children and adults may (or may not) possess (Hill 1997; Alderson 2000/2008; Christensen 2004; Christensen and James 2008b). They may be compounded by other assumptions based on gender, age, disability, ethnicity, language and culture. For example, the assumptions of some social workers regarding young children's lack of competence can exacerbate power imbalances because social workers might not believe that children can share their views or that, if they do, these views are unreliable and untrustworthy.

This can be further compounded by negative assumptions held about children with disabilities – an issue highlighted in a UN report, General Comment No. 9, that states, 'The Committee also notes that children with disabilities are still experiencing serious difficulties and [. . .] that the barrier is not the disability itself but rather a combination of social, cultural, attitudinal and physical obstacles which children with disabilities encounter in their daily lives (UN 2007: 2, para. 5).They often lead to a situation where differences between children and adults are exaggerated rather than the similarities that might exist between them, in terms of experience, for example, emphasized (Alderson 2000/2008). In the social worker–child relationships social workers have a legal mandate and it is hard to see, as outlined earlier, how and in what ways children can exercise choice and control, and how and in what ways power imbalances can be further addressed.

There are, however, a range of ways in which these power imbalances can be addressed. During the process of communication, for example, social workers need to be conscious of the varying roles that the social worker and the child can adopt. As will be seen in the case studies that are described later in this chapter, both the social worker and the child in their communication with each other variously adopted the roles of helper, instructor, advocate, interested person (Kortesluoma *et al.* 2003), learner (Christensen 2004) and/or observer. The adoption of and movement between these roles by the child and social worker alike serves to reduce power imbalances as a child, for example, is more likely to feel at ease if they perceive the social worker to be a helper or an interested person as opposed to a disinterested or distanced person.

Also, communication between children and social workers is more likely to 'flow' if the respective roles adopted by the child and the social workers are compatible and complementary. For example, in conversations when young children are using arts-based methods, they can adopt the role of instructor (asking the social worker to pass the sticky tape, cut material and write words down), and the social worker, in response, can adopt the role of helper in responding to their requests. Also, in relation to the narratives that accompanied the children's works they were doing, at certain points I took on the roles of learner and interested person while the children took on the role of teacher or narrator.

Another way of social workers addressing power imbalances is by paying attention to issues of their own presentation. Presentation encompasses a range of issues including, for example, dress, tone of voice, behaviour, gestures and eye contact. With regard to physical presentation when I was due to meet with young children to communicate with them I always carried an art box, rather than a briefcase or notepad and pen, with me. Through carrying the art box with me I hoped to convey a less formal and more approachable and fun image, conscious of the fact that first impressions do count. With regard to verbal presentation it is easy to fall into the trap of communicating in ways that are inaccessible to young children through the use of social work terminology and phrases. Explanations and information need to be short, concise, clear and accessible. It is also important to adopt a warm, kind and caring tone of voice and to greet children with a smile. In terms of other non-verbal communication, power imbalances can be addressed by being conscious of body language. A simple example includes not towering over children but crouching down so that eye contact is at the same level. These practical responses to addressing power imbalances are reflective of the principles of respect for each child, inclusivity (avoiding all patterns of pre-existing discrimination) and the adoption of a child-friendly approach (environment adapted to the capacities of the child) which, as outlined in the UN report on the right of a child to be heard (UN 2009: 27, paras (c), (e) and (f)), are integral to all processes that involve children.

Attention to boundaries

One final issue that should be mentioned is the importance of paying attention to boundaries in order to ensure that all practice is safe and sensitive to risk; a principle that should underpin all processes where children are involved and that acknowledges that, 'in certain situations, expression of views may involve risks. Adults have a responsibility towards the children with whom they work and must take every precaution to minimize the risk to children' (UN 2009: 27, para. (h)). For example, one role that children may assign to their social workers in the process of communication is that of therapist. This is not because the social worker has set himself or herself up as the trained therapist but because some young children can feel therapeutic release through the process of sharing memories, feelings and views (Butler and Williamson 1994). In the current research, and as was evident in the interview with Aine that provided the focus for the previous chapter, some young children may decide to use interviews to outwardly organize what had appeared to be internally jumbled up and unexpressed thoughts and feelings. Children's reluctance for the conversations to end (many of which may continue for well over an hour) appears to indicate that children feel they benefitted from the conversation.

Within this it is important for social workers to understand the limits, boundaries and parameters of their role and expertise and to achieve a balance. On the one hand, most social workers are not trained arts/play therapists and children may raise issues that require further exploration with a suitably qualified therapist with expertise in working with young children. However, and on the other hand, this should not detract from social workers establishing meaningful relationships and communicating with young children because each and every conversation can be beneficial for the child involved and carry deep meaning. A good illustration of this, while not relating to children as such, can be found in the work of the French sociologist Pierre Bourdieu. He conducted in-depth interviews with individuals in a community undergoing economic, political and social change. He found that interviewees engaged with the process of conversation about their feelings in a profound way. This led him to reflect:

> [C]ertain respondents, especially the most disadvantaged, seem to grasp this situation [of the research interview] as an exceptional opportunity offered to them to testify, to make themselves heard, to carry their experience over from the private to the public sphere; an opportunity also to *explain themselves* in the fullest sense of the term, that is, to construct their own point of view both about themselves and about the world and to bring into the open. It happens that, far from being simple instruments in the hands of the investigator, the respondents take over the interview themselves.
>
> (Bourdieu *et al.* 1999: 615, original emphasis)

The same is true of our conversations with children that can take on a deep significance. In a society where we spend only a small amount of time engaged in one-to-one conversations with young children it is not surprising that when the opportunity is offered it might be embraced by them as if it is the only opportunity they may have to communicate memories, perspectives and feelings. This should not make us fearful of these conversations but rather accept their value and to draw upon the expertise of others as/when necessary (Lefevre 2008).

Attention to boundaries also involves thinking about where to conduct conversations with young children. There is research that has considered the benefits and limitations of communicating with children at home as opposed to away from their own home (Bushin 2007; Punch 2007; Koprowska 2008: 636–66). However, ultimately, there is no one right answer and the decision that social workers make should be undertaken in conjunction with the child wherever possible and should take account of the issue to be discussed and the attitude of the main carers to the social worker's involvement, as well as the physical home environment and the child's own preferences, reactions and needs. For example, it may not be possible to build a relationship with a young child in their family home because the parents may continually interfere with the communication process or dominate it. The lack of respect for, or threat posed to, the social

---

EXERCISE
Imagine that you are about to begin a conversation with a young child who attends a pre-school nursery and try the following exercises:

- Think of the words you would use to tell a young child what the purpose of your meeting is with them, the issues that you are going to discuss and what will happen to the information.
- Think of the words you could use to tell a young child that if they talk about experiencing harm you cannot keep this confidential.
- Consider practical ways in which you have demonstrated (or could demonstrate) attention to power imbalances in your work with young children.

worker's role from parents can interfere with the social worker–child relationship and it may be better to see the child away from the family home.

Types of method

Having outlined the main issues that social workers need to take into account when communicating with young children the chapter will now consider some of the main methods used. In terms of the choice of method, Punch (2002b: 338) notes that

> [t]he choice of methods not only depends on the age, competence, experience, preference and social status of the research subjects but also on the cultural environment and the physical setting, as well as the research questions and the competencies of the researcher.

The current research used a variety of methods with children reflecting a combination of factors including the children's skills, my own skills and financial constraints. There were three main methods used: writing and drawing; playing, constructing and craftwork; and the creation of reality boxes. Each of these will now be considered in turn.

Writing and drawing

Some young children like to communicate through drawing and writing and these techniques have been used as a method for gaining the views of children for a long time. While these methods may seem straightforward enough, they have been criticized by Hill (1997) and Backett-Milburn and McKie (1999), among others, who argue that their uncritical use can reinforce negative stereotypes of young children as unable or unwilling to communicate. Furthermore, they suggest that the requirement for an 'expert adult' to reveal 'hidden meanings' in drawings further reinforces these stereotypes as it assumes that children are unable or unwilling to explain their own drawings. However, these criticisms draw attention to the underpinning views of children (as incompetent and immature) rather than being a critique of the method as such.

Reflecting an emphasis on the overarching themes of children's rights and social agency of young children, more recent research using this method has been informed by a view of young children as competent, creative and able to attribute their own meanings to their own constructions. Most recently this has been illustrated in the work of Coates and Coates (2006) and Einarsdottir *et al.* (2009) in which the drawings and writings of children have been accompanied by their own narratives that took place simultaneously to the drawing and writing being completed. This is rather different to getting children to 'explain' their work after its completion; a process which might evoke feelings in a child of being tested or having to produce meaning where there is none or giving meaning that is different to the meaning attributed during the process. The importance of accompanying narratives to children's drawing and writings is explained by Coates and Coates (2006: 221, 226) when they suggest that '[children's] simultaneous utterances might potentially inform the nature and content of the work and help elucidate their intentions and processes of thinking'.

In this chapter the case examples illustrate children's narratives as they are engaged in drawing and writing. Their engagement in these activities was either to represent a person, place, possession, view or feeling or as a means to control the intensity of the conversation because by focusing on what they were drawing or writing they were able to reduce eye contact with me, to distract the flow of the conversation and/or to change its direction. Within this it is important to respond to children's exercise of control and choice in a positive manner in order to avoid the process of communication becoming distressing or threatening. A number of examples of this will be provided in the next chapter.

Playing, constructing and craftwork

The second main method used in the current research with young children was playing, constructing and craftwork. All sorts of objects can be used, including soft toys, board games, sentence completion, use of music, dolls, puzzles, puppets and Lego (Crompton 1980; Lefevre 2008; McLeod 2008b). They can be used to establish rapport with a child before beginning a conversation around more specific issues. They can also be used to facilitate the process of communication through children and/or social workers appropriating the objects to represent people, places and possessions and enacting different scenarios. They can also be used to provide a visual map regarding family members and social networks.

I have found that even the simplest of things can be of great value in these activities. For example, I have an old tin of buttons and have used these to engage with children in the construction of a type of genogram where the buttons are used to help them depict who is who in their family and how close they feel to those identified people and pets. In this activity the child is invited to choose a button for each person in their social network, including themselves. A large piece of paper is also provided and the child is invited to place the button representing them in the centre of the page and then to place the other buttons around them, with those closest to them being those they like the most and those furthest away being those they least like. This activity can often generate a conversation about family and social networks. I have also used coins from my own purse for the same purpose.

As noted in the introduction, the emphasis is on the creative use of cheap materials to explore significant places, possessions, people and perspectives, and which, as will be discussed shortly, include the use of shoeboxes, 'end-of-line' craft materials such as scraps of card, pipe cleaners, stickers, buttons, wool and paints that can all be bought very cheaply. For some young children, as noted by Lefevre (2008: 131), their play represents 'the symbolic representation of experience' in which a child's internal world in terms of their thoughts, feelings and experiences 'will manifest itself in symbolic form through the infant's spontaneous play and can be communicated to others in this way'.

For other young children who use arts-based methods their actual constructions may not be a symbolic representation and, indeed, may bear no relationship at all to the issue being discussed. Rather, the process of the child engaging in art or craftwork and doing and talking at the same time, frees them up to explore their feelings because they can then use the material to control the depth, pace and content of the conversation. This was clearly evident, for example, in the discussions with Aine that were reported in the previous chapter. As with drawing and writing, the important aspect of practice when using this method is to concentrate on the narrative that the child shares as they are completing their work.

Reality boxes

The third and final main method that was used in the current research was 'reality boxes'. The concept of the reality box was inspired by an idea that I came across at the Childhoods 2005 Oslo Conference where young people involved in the opening ceremony of the conference had used small boxes to represent aspects of their identity and their perspectives. Essentially, and as I have come to adapt and use it in my own work, the reality box is an empty, undecorated shoebox with its lid. On the outside, children are invited to construct an image of themselves that best reflects how they come across to the outside world (their public person). In the inside they are invited to construct representations of their inner thoughts, feelings and perspectives (their private person). As with the drawings, the construction of the reality boxes were accompanied by the children's explanations of what they were making, what it means and why. Given that the young children's feelings in the current research had previously been left largely unexplored it was particularly important that it was the children's own words that accompanied the reality boxes rather than an imposed interpretation where there might have been the tendency, given the depth of the feelings typically expressed, to dilute, sanitize, reinterpret and/or misinterpret the meaning that the child wished to convey. This can be seen in the previous chapter where it was important that Aine attributed her own explanations to her work and her choice of stickers and art materials.

Using multiple methods

Overall the uses of writing, drawing, craftwork and reality boxes were all methods available simultaneously in the current research. Of course it is possible to combine these methods in order to piece together information from a wide range of sources to build up a comprehensive picture. This is precisely the underlying philosophy of the Mosaic approach developed by Clark and Moss (2001) which is a framework that has been developed to gain the perspectives of young children in early childhood settings by piecing together – like a mosaic – information from a variety of sources including: researchers' observations of the children; interviews with children, parents and practitioners; children undertaking tours of their setting; children taking photographs; and researchers making maps/books with them. While not used directly in the current research, Clark and Statham (2005: 52) discuss how this approach could be very appropriate for social workers working with young children, stating that,

> [i]n particular, the approach could help children to reflect on their own experiences, provide a bridge for children and adults to discuss meanings together, and contribute to future decision-making.

Specific examples could include helping young children prepare for placement moves, ascertaining the different perspectives and priorities of siblings placed in care and engaging foster carers in the process of understanding the impact of transition from a young child's point of view. For example, Clark and Statham (2005) discuss how children could be involved in making photograph albums and life storybooks showing their former families as part of their transition to a new family.

Summary

This chapter has considered the use of participatory methods in communication with young children. It has highlighted that, within a child rights-based framework, there are a number of issues that social workers need to acknowledge and address in using these methods with young children. These include the requirement for social workers to pay attention to ethical issues, power imbalances and boundaries in their relationships with young children. They also include the requirement for social workers to respect the freedoms and choices of young children, to respect their individuality and to respect their views and feelings. The chapter then moved on to consider some of the main methods used in communication with young children. The main issue for social workers is not so much their knowledge of these methods but rather the nuts and bolts of how they actually work in practice. What does a conversation with a young child look like? What happens during the process of the conversation? What methods are used? How exactly do they help? These are all issues considered in the next chapter, which uses a number of detailed case studies, involving real-life conversations, with young children ages 4–7 years, in order to provide a detailed illustration of the practicalities and realities of using these methods in practice.

EXERCISE
- Have you had any experience in communicating with children either professionally or personally?
- Have you used any methods to help you communicate with children?
- Which of these methods would you feel most/least comfortable with?
- Do you think that there are certain types of method that might work better than others?

7 Communicating with young children

Case studies

Summary of chapter content

The purpose of this chapter is to illustrate skills and methods in action through the use of three in-depth case studies. The case studies are all based on real-life excerpts of detailed conversations with young children between the ages of 4 and 7 years. The case studies have been selected to illustrate the different ways in which children use methods to explore their memories, feelings and views about their families and about life since they have come into care. The case studies also illustrate all of the key principles and practice points outlined in the previous chapter.

Introduction

As stated in the previous chapter, one of the best ways of understanding how methods can be used in communicating with young children is through real-life case examples. This chapter considers how the various methods outlined in the previous chapters, and principles underpinning them, have been used in practice in conversations with three children: Grady (aged 4 years), Ben (aged 5 years) and Finn (aged 7 years). Using detailed excerpts of conversations with these three children, the chapter illustrates the use of a range of methods in ascertaining their knowledge, perspectives and feelings about their family lives, the reasons for their removal from their family homes and their views on their current care circumstances. Before turning to the first case study, however, it is important to take a step back and consider briefly some of the key ethical issues associated with this type of research.

Ethical issues

The initial framework for and design of the current research addressed a number of ethical issues prior to commencing. These reflect UN General Comment No. 12 (*The Right of the Child to be Heard*) (UN 2009), which, as noted in Chapter Four, states that involving children should be transparent, informative, respectful, voluntary, child-friendly, safe and sensitive to risk and accountable. With regard to being transparent and informative, information packs were supplied to all participants selected to be involved (children, parents and social workers) regarding the purpose, content and aims of the research. In order to be child-friendly, appropriate information sheets were designed that were colourful and attractive and were prepared for the children to be read through with an adult. In order to ensure that involvement was voluntary, informed consent was secured individually from the parents, children and their social workers to be involved in individual, in-depth interviews and to use the findings to write reports with the aim of helping social workers improve their practice.

Because of the status of the young children (they were in state care and the subject of legal orders whereby legal parental responsibility is shared by both social services and the birth parents) consent was also defined as a three-way process involving the child, the parent and social services. This meant in practice that if any party did not consent then that particular case study would not be included. Consent was also defined as an ongoing process based on the clear understanding that anyone could make a choice to withdraw at any time in the process. If anyone chose to withdraw his or her data would no longer be used. This was made clear in the information provided and during the course of the individual interviews. Through these mechanisms the research process aimed to address issues of safety and risk.

Further mechanisms to address issues of safety and risk included the provision of clear information regarding the constraints around confidentiality. It was explained, in line with child protection procedures, that if children revealed harm they had suffered or might suffer, social services were alerted. Other than that, confidentiality was guaranteed and all data (verbal, non-verbal and arts-based) were anonymized. Discussions took place with children as part of my conversations with them about whether they would be happy for their artwork to be included in work that I was planning to prepare to help improve social work practice and thus whether they were happy for me to take photographs of their artwork to show others.

As indicated in earlier chapters, there was a range of responses from the children from not wanting their work photographed to those who did and also from those who actually wanted to put their name on their work to those who were keen to ensure that their anonymity was secure. Others wanted me to store and keep their work whereas others wished to take it home with them, with or without photographs having been taken. These wishes were all honoured and were indicative of the respectful approach adopted throughout the research towards the children. Finally, named people were identified prior to the conversations to act as a support in the event that this was needed.

Even with all these safeguards in place, questions could still be raised regarding whether the children in particular, and maybe adults as well, really knew what they were getting involved in and thus what they were letting themselves in for. In one sense, the answer to this is 'no', in that it was not possible to be prescriptive about what they might raise in their conversations, what effect it might have on them or specifically how their information would be used (in terms of the specific detail of training events, books and reports). In another sense, however, the answer is 'yes', in that they were all aware of the broad issues to be explored, the fact that their perspectives would be used to help other social workers in their practice and that this might involve training and writing. Where possible children were informed as to how their information would be used.

Grady (aged 4 years): use of shoeboxes

Background information

The first case study to be explored is Grady, one of six children. He had been known to social services since he was about 2 years old. He lived in a family where there had been concerns regarding parental alcohol/drug misuse, domestic violence and abuse, debt and frequent house moves. There were several occasions when the social worker was concerned that Grady's mother seemed to be under the influence of an unidentified substance that caused slurred speech and dilated pupils. Grady's mother experienced violence in her relationships with partners (past and present) that, on occasion, led to her suffering physical injuries. House moves tended to be unplanned, leaving behind unpaid bills amounting to thousands of pounds.

The children often arrived at school late, unfed, ill-prepared with no bags, no books and no snacks for break time and sometimes they were inappropriately dressed, notably coming to school with no coats in winter. The children's health needs were not attended to and appointments with speech and language therapists, the eye clinic and the ear, nose and throat clinic were missed on numerous occasions. For some of the children their unmet health needs affected their progress at school because hearing and sight difficulties made it impossible to engage fully in class work. The children's physical living conditions at home were chaotic, with social workers reporting big piles of unwashed clothes, dirty plates and half-eaten food strewn throughout. Bedrooms were found to have bare (and in some instances urine-sodden) mattresses and sparse furnishings. Some of the children had witnessed incidents of domestic violence and been threatened themselves during the course of these incidents. Given the cumulative concerns the children were eventually removed from their family home. Grady was separated from his siblings and placed with foster carers.

At the time of my conversation with Grady he had been living with foster carers for several months and was seeing his family members on a weekly basis but supervised by social services. Attempts to rehabilitate him home were ongoing but facing difficulties because of his mother's failure to regularly attend parenting-skills appointments that were identified as a necessary element of the plan to return Grady home. The purpose of my conversation with Grady was to explore his understanding of the reasons he was in care, to ascertain his feelings and perspectives about his family and his life in care. The conversation took place in a room in a social services building that had a low coffee table in it.

Beginning of conversation

To begin with, I had laid out some of the materials on a coffee table before Grady came into the room. The intention was that if he wished to use the materials I would sit on the floor next to the table while he stood by the table (making us more or less the same height as each other). This is a practical way in which to address the issue of the power imbalances that are present in a conversation between a social worker and a child. When he entered the room Grady went straight to the table and started picking up various craft materials. My aim at the start was to make him as comfortable as possible and I began by thanking him and asking if he would like to take his jacket off and the initial conversation continued as follows:

Grady: It's sparkly [*referring to a tube of coloured glitter glue*].
KW: It's sparkly. Thank you very much, Grady, for coming to see me. I was going to have a chat with you today about all the people that you know. Would that be OK?
Grady: [*Nods head.*]

KW:	Yeah? Wow [*responding to Grady showing KW a glitter pen he has picked up*]! Now.
Grady:	Gina's [*pointing to a scarf belonging to his carer's daughter that he has borrowed*].
KW:	That's Gina's, is it?
Grady:	Aha.
KW:	Let's see if we can get some more, would you like to take your wee jacket off, 'cause I think it'll be quite warm in here. That's it. There [*encouraging Grady as he takes off his jacket*].
Grady:	I'm warm.
KW:	Aha.
Grady:	Got too warm.

Encouraging Grady to take his coat off and letting him feel at ease with the materials on the coffee table are examples of establishing the right conditions for the conversation to proceed, which as noted in Chapter Five, are important issues to attend to during the beginnings stage of the conversation and illustrate a respectful approach towards Grady.

Exploring Grady's knowledge about his home circumstances

Having made Grady comfortable he began to go through the craft materials on the table. What cannot be shown in the transcripts and yet was a feature throughout our conversation was my tone of voice, which was gentle, warm and affirming and my facial expression, which was relaxed and open. The conversation proceeded, where it left off, as follows:

KW:	Now, do you want to give me your jacket? [*Grady looks at his jacket and hands it to KW*] There, we'll hang it up on the door. There, that's a good boy.
Grady:	[*Begins to play with paper and the shoeboxes. KW watches in silence for a while.*]
KW:	Let's have a look. Oh, that's good [*referring to a shoebox that Grady has picked up, turned over and put material on. More silence as KW watches Grady*]. Grady can you tell me where you're living at the moment?
Grady:	Here [*referring to shoebox*].
KW:	In this house? Whose is that house [*referring to a second box Grady has picked up*]?
Grady:	Where's my box? Where's my box [*referring to the first box he has put on the floor behind him*]?
KW:	Where's your box? Oh, here.
Grady:	It can be mummy's house.
KW:	That's mummy's house? OK. There's mummy's house. And who else lives in mummy's house?
Grady:	Everybody else.

Grady selected three shoeboxes to represent the homes of his family, foster carers and respite carers (see Figure 7.1). Unlike my work with Aine, I did not guide Grady as

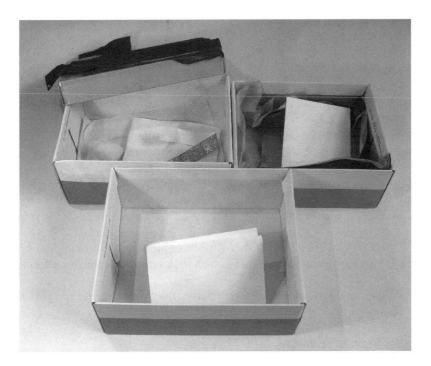

Figure 7.1 The inside of Grady's three houses.

to how I thought he might use the shoeboxes. Rather, he selected the boxes himself to represent houses. Supporting his use of the shoeboxes in this way is an example of respecting Grady's individuality and his freedoms and choices, two of the important principles that underpin a child rights-based approach to the use of participatory methods as discussed in Chapter Six.

Our conversation began, using the shoeboxes selected by Grady to represent houses, with an exploration as to what Grady did in each house:

KW:	Yes, it opens, it's glitter [. . .] Which house are you decorating with the glitter?
Grady:	All of them.
KW:	All of them? And what kind of things do you do at Giselle's [respite carer] house?
Grady:	Play with the Lego.
KW:	Play with the Lego?
Grady:	The Lego man.
KW:	And the Lego man?
Grady:	And play things with the Lego.
KW:	And play things with the Lego? And what do you do at mummy's house?
Grady:	Play on the bike.
KW:	You play on the bike?
Grady:	Oh wow! Two pens!

KW: Yes, it's two pens in one. And then what do you do at Gordon's [foster-father] house? See, if you put some glue on and you put the glitter on top . . . [*Silence as KW watches Grady use glue and glitter.*] And what do you do at Gordon's house? Can you remember?
Grady: Play.
KW: You play as well? So you've got three houses that you play in?
Grady: Yes.

This aspect of the conversation shows the use of listening, questioning and responding skills, which were outlined and discussed in detail in Chapter Five. It can be seen that most of the questions are closed questions resulting in Grady providing short answers. It can also be seen that, in terms of responding skills, the skill of reflecting back is the one mainly used. The shoeboxes provided a method through which Grady's views about his circumstances could be explored further as illustrated below:

KW: And do you know why you don't live at mummy's house anymore?
Grady: Because my mummy, mummy don't look after, mummy don't look after us properly.
KW: Mummy don't [*using same word as Grady for symmetry in the interview process*] look after you's properly?
Grady: Aha.
KW: What kind of things?
Grady: Us!
KW: Mummy didn't look after you properly?
Grady: Yeah [. . .] [*Silence. Grady cuts out some paper.*]
KW: That's lovely. Are you going to put that on the house or is that just going to be your picture?
Grady: I'm going to [*doesn't finish sentence but earnestly concentrates on boxes. More silence. Grady then looks at KW.*] . . .
KW: Grady, you see when you say to me that mummy didn't look after you properly, what do you mean? Did she feed you?
Grady: No.
KW: No?
Grady: No.
KW: Did she put clean clothes on you?
Grady: Yes.
KW: But she didn't feed you?
Grady: No.
KW: Were you always hungry?
Grady: Yeah, my stomach was rumbling.
KW: Your stomach was rumbling? And . . .
Grady: Sometimes mummy would sometimes give food.
KW: Sometimes she gave you food?
Grady: Yeah [*more cutting of paper*].
KW: And sometimes she didn't? And was your house warm or cold?
Grady: Warm.
KW: Your house was nice and warm? So she kept you warm but she didn't feed you all the time?

Grady:	No and . . .
KW:	And?
Grady:	It's a bit difficult [*referring to family home he is making but also appeared to be an indication that the content of the conversation was difficult because of his faltering eye contact and voice tailing off*].
KW:	Yes, it's a bit difficult.

It can be seen that this part of the conversation involved a number of skills. In terms of listening skills there were non-verbal messages from Grady at different points in the conversation where Grady diverted his attention from the conversation to the shoeboxes. This was used as time out from the conversation. I only continued with the conversation when Grady made eye contact with me again using a warm and gentle tone of voice. This reflects a respectful approach towards Grady, a principle discussed in Chapters Four, Five and Six. With regard to questioning skills, most of the questions I asked were closed questions. While this elicited information from Grady, in retrospect it might have been better to use some more open questions. However, the use of open-ended questions too early in the process also risked him feeling vulnerable or maybe that he was engaged in some kind of test. In terms of responding skills there are a few examples of where the skills of summarizing and reflecting back were used to indicate to Grady that I was hearing everything he was saying.

One last interesting point to also note is that Grady said his house was 'warm' and in response I said 'nice and warm'. While this was a colloquialism on my part it was, with hindsight, probably a mistake as it could have deterred Grady from further discussion about his house because he did not say it was nice and yet I had. From here the conversation moved on to explore with Grady his understanding and experience of being removed from his family home:

KW:	OK, oh, right, we've got to do those ones as well. OK [*referring to pictures Grady is completing while talking*]. And who took you from your mummy's house to Gwendolyn's [foster carer] house?
Grady:	A social worker.
KW:	A social worker? And do you know why she took you away from your mummy's house?
Grady:	No.
KW:	No? And how did you feel when she took you from your mummy's house?
Grady:	Happy.
KW:	You felt happy? Did you not want to stay with your mummy?
Grady:	Yeah.
KW:	You did? So did that make you feel happy or sad?
Grady:	Sad.
KW:	You were sad? And did you know why they took you to a different house?
Grady:	No [*pause while Grady draws figures on paper*].
KW:	No? Did anyone say to you why you were moving?
Grady:	No.

One aspect of this conversation that stands out is my response to Grady saying he was happy when he was removed. I had not anticipated that response as I had assumed he would be sad. This had an impact on my subsequent questions because, as noted above, I did not ask Grady why he was happy (which would, in retrospect, have been a very useful question) but did pursue questions about him feeling sad. This is a good example of the influence that assumptions can have on the content and direction of conversations and a good example of what should be avoided in practice. It shows how power imbalances can work in subtle ways with, in this instance, my own, adult assumptions leading the conversation in a particular direction. Had I managed to keep these in check the conversation might have gone in a different direction.

Another of the aspects of this part of the conversation that is striking is that while Grady had memories about some experiences at home of not being fed (and, as seen later, of observing parental arguments that left him feeling afraid) he did not make the link between those and the reasons why he was removed from home. To social workers it might have seemed obvious that it was the concerns about his mother's care of him (lack of food being one of these concerns) that led to his removal. However, for Grady this was not obvious; instead, he was confused. He also indicated that he did not recall having any information about why he was being removed from his mother's care at the time of those events.

Exploring Grady's feelings

In the above conversation with Grady it was seen that he expressed his feelings of happiness and sadness. He explored these feelings further when making his family home (see Figure 7.2) and drawing all the people who lived inside the family home (see Figure 7.3). One example of this was when he recalled an argument between his stepfather and mother:

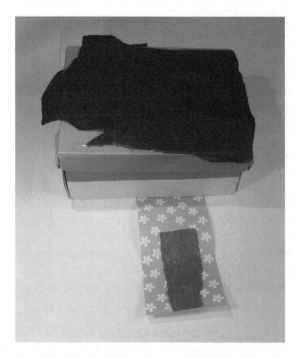

Figure 7.2 The outside of Grady's family home.

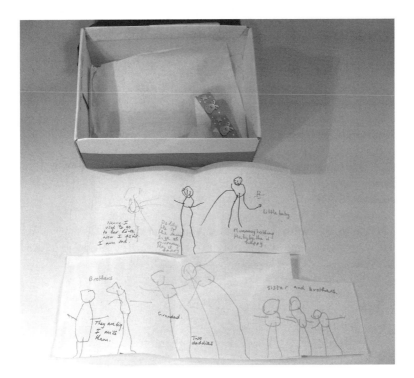

Figure 7.3 The inside of Grady's family home.

KW: And [. . .] you said before that you remember that your mummy and Gerard [stepfather] had an argument?

Grady: Yes.

KW: Yes? What happened in that argument?

Grady: Got afraid.

KW: Aha?

Grady: Shaky. Got shaky.

KW: Yeah, you got shaky?

However, and in contrast, he also said the following when describing his stepfather, who he was drawing at the time:

KW: And what about Gerard? What was he like?

Grady: Nice and awesome.

KW: He was nice and awesome? Aww!

Grady: Is there any more [*referring to glitter pens*]?

KW: Yes. Right, that's it. Oh, that's a nice colour isn't it?

Grady: And you get [*stops to pick up glue*].

When Grady was drawing all the people who lived in his family home I invited him to reflect on his feelings about his family:

KW:	Right. And is this house a happy house where all these people live?
Grady:	It was [*drawing mum and Gerard on paper*].
KW:	This used to be a happy house?
Grady:	Yeah. And now it isn't.
KW:	And now it isn't? Why is it not happy anymore?
Grady:	'Cause we don't live with mummy and Gerard.

These feelings were further reinforced when he described his feelings about his nanny (maternal grandmother):

KW:	Oh, there's some room there. Who else do you want to put on there? Let's move that back.
Grady:	Nanny.
KW:	Nanny?
Grady:	Nanny is the same size as mummy and Gerard.
KW:	Nanny is the same size as mummy and Gerard? And do you like nanny?
Grady:	Yeah.
KW:	Did you used to go to nanny's house?
Grady:	Yeah.
KW:	Yeah?
Grady:	But now I don't.
KW:	Now you don't? And how do you feel about that?
Grady:	Sad.

In this part of the conversation it can be seen that Grady identified feelings of sadness, fear and happiness. He also was able to explore the fact that while he had been scared when witnessing an argument between his mother and stepfather he also felt that his stepfather was 'nice and awesome'. This was an extremely important part of the conversation with Grady in that, in all of the forms that accompanied his move into care and the subsequent planning and decision-making around his care, there was absolutely no mention of his own feelings at all. This is despite the fact that, as noted in Chapters Two and Four, social workers are now legally mandated to ascertain the wishes and feelings of children and to be creative in the ways they attempt to do this.

The conversation with Grady about his feelings does raise the issue of needing to be aware of boundaries for the following reasons. First, when children start to explore their feelings the social worker may feel those feelings too. The social worker needs to acknowledge the child's feelings, be aware of their own emotional responses and ensure that their responses do not interfere with the process of the conversation, as discussed at length in Chapter Five when exploring the conversation with Aine. Second, while the social worker may hear about children's feelings they may not be the best placed to work through some of their more deep-seated and unresolved feelings. It is important for social workers to acknowledge the limits of their own expertise and professional role and to call on the help of others as/when necessary.

Exploring Grady's views

In addition to exploring Grady's memories of home, his understanding of the reasons he was in care and his feelings about this, the purpose of the conversation was also to ascertain his views about his current care circumstances. Grady uses the shoeboxes and some coloured pom-poms (small, coloured fluffy balls) to explore his views about his relationships with his current carers and his future:

KW: There it is. OK. There's your people. There they all are [. . .] There's another green one, there's two blue ones, there's three blue ones [*referring to coloured pom-pom balls that Grady has chosen to represent people in his network*].
Grady: Give us another green one [*referring to a pom-pom ball*].
KW: There.
Grady: But where is the other one [*referring to a pom-pom ball*]?
KW: [. . .] I think that's all there is, you can check in that box over there.
KW: [*Silence while KW watches Grady engaged in play.*] Grady, where would you like to live in the future?
Grady: All of them.
KW: All of them? Would you?
Grady: Aha. But I can't.
KW: All of them? But you can't?
Grady: Put the, all the, put all the houses together, put them altogether.
KW: Put them all together?
Grady: All of them, all the houses together.

Grady's symbolic resolution to the question as to where he might live in the future was to stick the shoebox houses of his mother, respite carer and foster carer together as one big house complex. Because Grady's solution was not realistic in the sense that he could never live with all of these people in one big house then it is easy to dismiss his opinion as confused. However, if time is taken to draw out what the underlying message might be (e.g. 'these people are all important to me and I would like to retain my relationships with all of them'), then Grady's opinions are understandable, more realistic and would probably reflect the views of many others if they found themselves in a similar position.

In summary, Grady shared some of his experiences of living at home. He recalled that he was not always fed and that on those occasions he felt hungry. He also said that he felt afraid when he saw/heard an argument between his mother and his stepfather but that his stepfather was also 'nice and awesome'. He remembered when he was removed from his mother's care and that he felt happy and sad about this. However, at the time he was being removed he did not know why this was happening. Grady had feelings of sadness when thinking about his family home and some of the significant people he left behind. Having said this he also had feelings of happiness in relation to the relationships with his foster carers and respite carers. His view was that all of these people were significant to him and that he wished to retain his contact with all of these people in the future.

The summary above serves as an example of what could be included in social services reports (for meetings and court) regarding the wishes and feelings of young children. In those reports there is a section, to be completed by the social worker, set aside for outlining the wishes and feelings of the child concerned. Where possible the actual words of the child, or excerpts of the conversation, should be included.

EXERCISE
- Re-read the conversations above and find examples of:
  — closed question(s)
  — open question(s)
  — summarizing/reflecting back
  — mirroring.
- What principles underpin the use of the method (shoeboxes) in this conversation?
- Looking at the conversations, what could have been done better and why?
- What are the main issues that have emerged from the conversation with Grady?
- List some practical ways in which you could ensure that Grady's views were fully and accurately presented in a report for court or a review meeting.
- What do you think might be the response/reaction from parents and/or professionals to these views?
- What could you do to address these responses/reactions?

Ben (aged 5 years): use of props and craftwork

Background information

Ben, the focus for this second case study, is one of three children. His family had been known to social services for a number of years before he was even born. There were concerns regarding parental alcohol dependency, in relation to both his mother and her then partner. For example, social services and the police had found Ben's mother highly intoxicated while caring for her children on more than one occasion. Furthermore, there were significant concerns regarding domestic violence and abuse where there had been several police call-outs to the family home, injuries to Ben's mother requiring hospital treatment, and instigation of civil proceedings by Ben's mother to obtain injunctions against her partner that were then breached by the partner. Lastly, the family had moved home on several occasions in an unplanned manner following allegations of intimidation by people with paramilitary connections.

The children were removed from home following incidents of physical and emotional abuse. In relation to physical abuse there were concerns regarding over-chastisement and unexplained injuries to the head and body of one of the children. With regard to emotional abuse, the children were exposed to repeated incidents of domestic violence and abuse that had left them anxious, unable to sleep and unable to concentrate in school. When the three children (Bonnie, Ben and Bella) were removed from home Bonnie was placed with foster carers. Bella and Ben were placed together for a short time in foster care and then moved and placed in different foster homes. The purpose of my interview with Ben was to explore his knowledge, experiences and feelings about his home life, the reason why he was in care and his feelings about his current and future care circumstances. The interview took place in a room at a social services office. The room had a large meeting table with chairs. I had taken the opportunity before the meeting to put out some of the art materials on the table.

Beginning of conversation

Ben entered the room having been shown around the social services building, which, although familiar to him, he wanted to tour again. Respecting Ben's individuality was an important principle underpinning the start of our conversation with each other. Throughout the conversation my tone of voice was gentle, warm and affirming. At times we laughed together, especially when, as seen later, Ben talks about one of the problems with his pet guinea pig. The conversation began as follows:

KW: That's great [*reference to Ben sitting down on a chair next to KW to start conversation*].
Ben: Ooh! I can't open this [*referring to tube of coloured glitter glue*].
KW: Do you remember you said you'd try and help me understand a few things?
Ben: Aha.
KW: Well, can I ask you some questions and you see if you can help me with the answers?
Ben: Yes.
KW: Great. So I can understand a wee bit about you.

It can be seen at the start of the conversation that there was clarification about the purpose of the conversation and that, as in the case of Grady, having some art materials laid out prior to Ben entering the room was to help him feel at ease by having something to focus on as he settled down. In the beginning of the interview Ben identified who lived in his family by listing them. The conversation moved on to exploring with Ben why he thought he no longer lived at home:

KW: Do you know why you're living with Belinda and Bill [foster carers]?
Ben: Aha.
KW: Why are you living there?
Ben: 'Cause I don't want to live with my auntie [ex-foster carer].
KW: You don't want to live with your auntie? And what's your auntie's name?
Ben: I don't know.
KW: Oh.
Ben: Nanny and Bernard [partner of the auntie].
KW: Oh yes, you don't, why don't you want to live with them?
Ben: I wish you had a roller thing [*referring to a rolling pin that he would like to use to roll out playdough*].
KW: Yeah, I might have to use my hands. Shall we try?
Ben: Aha. [*Time passes as we roll playdough with our hands into a long snake. KW waits for Ben to re-engage through eye contact.*]
KW: Why don't you want to live with Bridget and Bernard?
Ben: Do you have a roller?

This conversation with Ben illustrates how Ben used playdough to distract and deflect attention away from the conversation about why he no longer wanted to live with his ex-foster carers. Ben did not answer my questions or look at me. I interpreted Ben's reaction as a coping mechanism and as a way of him saying, 'I don't want to talk about this'. After allowing time to pass, and attempting to pick up the conversation once more, this aspect of the conversation moved on because Ben did not want to talk about this issue anymore. This approach shows a respect for Ben's right not to express his views and a respect for his choices.

Exploring Ben's feelings

One of the themes that emerges in the following conversation with Ben is that he chose to use objects in the room as props, rather than the methods I had brought with me, to explore his relationship with, and feelings about, his mother. During this aspect of the conversation Ben was also very mobile, jumping to different parts of what was a fairly large room while continuing his conversation with me. I supported Ben in these choices by not interfering with his choices or trying to redirect his attention. These are other practical ways in which I attempted to respect Ben's individuality, choices and his preferences as outlined in Chapter Six and that are reflective of some of the key principles characterizing a child rights-based approach that should underpin the use of participatory methods.

When using a spare, unplugged phone that Ben found on a shelf and that he used to conduct 'pretend' conversations, Ben revealed that he had previously hit his mother and that he had been bad because of this.

KW: And you're going to phone [*referring to Ben picking up a spare, unplugged phone in the room that he found on a bookshelf*]?
Ben: Yes.
KW: Right. Hold on.
Ben: Bring the phone over here.
KW: The telephone's just on its way Ben.
Ben: Hmm?
KW: The telephone's just on its way.
Ben: Oh right.
KW: Ben are you wanting to phone me?
Ben: Aha. Hello.
KW: Hello Ben. How are you?
Ben: How are you doing?
KW: I'm fine thanks. How are you?
Ben: Alright.
KW: Great.
Ben: You're being bad [*talking to KW as if KW is Ben, as indicated by Ben pointing to him and then KW*].
KW: I'm being bad? Oh dear. What have I done wrong?
Ben: You've hit mummy [*talking to KW as if KW is Ben*].
KW: Oh dear, oh dear [. . .] Did I hit mummy?
Ben: Aha.
KW: Dear goodness.
Ben: Say sorry.
KW: [. . .] Oh. Sorry!
Ben: Bye then.
KW: Bye!

Ben used both the telephone and me (in an acting role playing the part of Ben) to explore an event in which he had hit his mother and how he had said sorry about this. His use of me in this capacity is an example of our changing roles within the conversation. In this part of the conversation Ben took on the role of 'person in charge' and I acquired the role of 'Ben'. This is an example, as outlined in Chapter Six, of ways in which the power imbalances within a conversation can be addressed through adopting different roles or by role reversal.

In the conversation below Ben used a computer that was also present in the room but not part of the materials I had brought along, to express his feelings about his 'missing' mother who was missing in the sense of Ben not being with her and not knowing precisely where she was:

KW:　　Right, are you trying something [*watching Ben playing with a computer in the room which is on 'close down' but not closed down completely*]?

Ben:　　Doing this [*indicating the computer*].

KW:　　Who are you typing a letter to?

Ben:　　Mummy.

KW:　　And what are you saying in there?

Ben:　　[*Mumbles*] Where are you?

KW:　　What are you saying to your mummy?

Ben:　　[*Mumbles*] Are you there?

KW:　　[. . .] And what else are you saying to your mummy?

Ben:　　[*Mumbles*] Are you there?

Ben then went back to the telephone:

KW:　　Who is the most favourite person that you want to phone?

Ben:　　Oh. Mummy!

KW:　　Aha. Which mummy?

Ben:　　Beryl [birth mother]

KW:　　[*Later in interview, talking to Ben who has phone in his hand*] What do you want to say?

Ben:　　Hello! Hello! Mummy! Come and get me.

Ben's use of props helped him to explore his relationship with, and his feelings about, his mother. During the next part of the conversation Ben then used art materials to make his mother several 'presents' as he described them. What was revealing, in his use of methods, as shown in the remainder of this section, was the intensity and consistency of his feelings towards his mother given that, at the point the research was undertaken, he had been living away from his mother for over two years.

As shown in Figure 7.4, he made his mother an Indian carefully laid out and stuck on paper for safekeeping.

KW:　　I love what you've made there!

Ben:　　It's very good.

KW:　　Yeah, who is it?

Ben:　　It's an Indian.

KW:　　It's an Indian?

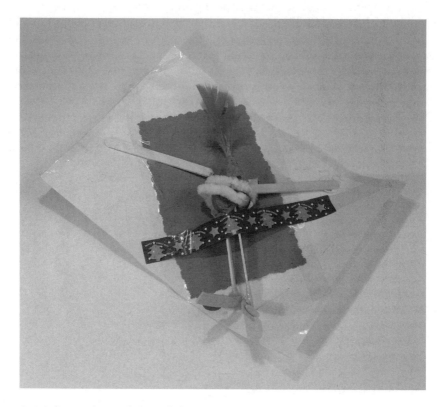

Figure 7.4 A figure of an Indian made by Ben for his mother.

Ben:	Like.
KW:	And has the Indian got a name?
Ben:	No.
KW:	No? You're not calling?
Ben:	[*Interrupts*] My mummy can make one.
KW:	Your mummy can make a name for it? Is it a girl or a boy?
Ben:	It's a [*inaudible*].
KW:	A boy?
Ben:	A girl.
KW:	It's a girl? So your mummy's got to think of a name?
Ben:	I know, give her my guinea pig's name.
KW:	What's your guinea pig's, what's your?
Ben:	Buster.
KW:	And what colour is your guinea pig?
Ben:	Brown. Do you know what she does? She poos on my hands sometimes!
KW:	Ooh! [*KW and Ben laugh together.*]

Ben also used the available methods to make further presents for his mummy, including an elephant and a picture of his mother with his sister, as can be seen in Figures 7.5 and 7.6.

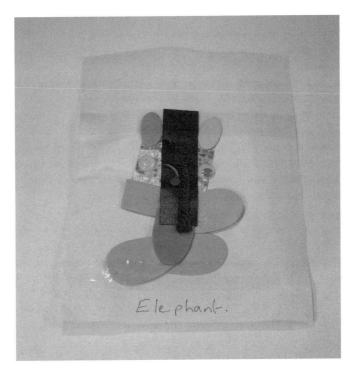

Figure 7.5 A figure of an elephant made by Ben for his mother.

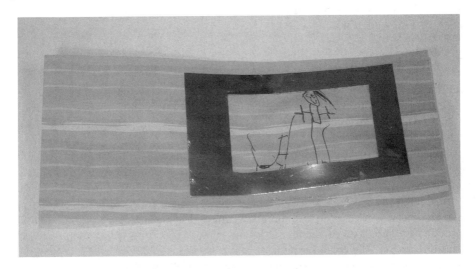

Figure 7.6 A picture of mum and baby sister made by Ben.

Ben: I'll draw my mummy.
KW: Great. That's nice. And what's your mummy doing?
Ben: With Bria.
KW: She's with Bria? And what does Bria look like?

Ben:	She, she has to go in a buggy.

Ben: She, she has to go in a buggy.
KW: Bria goes in a buggy?
Ben: Why did they have to call it a buggy, 'cause that?
KW: Yes, what do you think buggy means?
Ben: It's a pram.
Ben: [. . .] Are we going to make more presents for my mummy?
KW: That'll be very nice.
Ben: She's getting loads.

By the end of the interview Ben had made a puppet, an elephant and drawings as, in his words, presents for his mother, stating that 'she is going to get loads'.

During the course of the conversation Ben also expressed his sadness that his contact with his mother did not happen as often as he would like:

KW: OK. So, Ben, there's a few [other] things that I just want to talk about today.
Ben: Why am I not going to get to see my mummy?
KW: Why are you not going to get to see your mummy? Yes, that's one of the things I was going to talk about. Aren't you seeing her today?
Ben: Yeah, but why will I not get to see her all them days, two days?
KW: Oh yes. Well, that's a good question. I don't know. Why do you think that you are not?
Ben: 'Cause, hmm don't know.
KW: You don't know? And how does it make you feel when you don't get to see her?
Ben: Don't know. A bit sad.
KW: A bit sad? OK.
Ben: Yeah.
KW: Right. OK.

It can be seen in the conversation above that Ben asked a very specific question regarding the days that he could not see his mother. I did not know the answer to this and yet Ben had a right to receive information to help him understand decisions made about his contact with his mother. This appeared particularly pertinent given his apparent unresolved feelings about his mother. In discussion with Ben I told him that I thought it might be useful if he spoke to someone about his feelings some more and that maybe his social worker could help answer his questions about contact. We agreed that I should let his social worker know about this issue, which later I did. This was not surprising to the social worker who had already requested some specialist help for Ben. The approach here shows an awareness of boundaries, to the limits of my own role and of the need to respect the role of others.

Throughout the process of exploring his feelings with him Ben was very active in his engagement with a range of methods to explore and express his feelings, which were child-centred and reflected Ben's own capacities. This, as noted in Chapters Five and Six, is an important principle underpinning the involvement of children in any process. Some social workers might think that the more props and materials there are in a room, the more these might act as a distraction to the process of a conversation. This might sometimes be the case. However, for Ben, far from it being a distraction, the variety offered by both the room and the materials in the room facilitated and supported his exploration of his feelings. Again these issues show respect for the individuality and capacities of Ben but also an acknowledgement that they might not suit all children.

Exploring Ben's views

In addition to using props and art materials, Ben also engaged in conversation where he expressed his view, in the following conversation, that he would like to return to his mother's care:

KW: And do you want to move to a new place, Ben?

Ben: Yeah.

KW: You do want to move? Why do you want to move from Belinda and Bill [foster carers]?

Ben: 'Cause I love my mummy.

KW: Because you love your mummy?

Ben: Aha.

KW: But if you move from Belinda and Bill, does that mean you're going back to mummy or you're going to a new family?

Ben: Back to mummy.

KW: Ah. So you want to go from Belinda and Bill back to mummy? What happens if you have to move to another new family?

Ben: Don't know. If I get to, to move, I have to, can then go back to them and then if I get a new family I can go back to them and if I get another family I can go back to them and get back to mummy.

KW: Is that what you want to do?

Ben: Yeah.

KW: Yes? You're, so even if you keep moving from family to family, what you want to do is go back to your mummy?

Ben: Yeah.

In reality Ben could not return home because a court had determined that it was not in his best interests to do so. Ben's unresolved feelings about his mother and why he could no longer live with her were therefore a painful testament of what he felt he had lost and what he could not ever fully recover. His deeply held feelings, as stated above, do raise the issue of paying attention to boundaries. I was not having a conversation with Ben in a therapeutic context and yet Ben was revealing important information regarding his feelings that might require further help by a trained therapist. As stated above his social worker was informed of this but, as already stated, was aware of these issues and had already referred him for specialist help.

Finn (aged 7 years): use of art materials

Background information

Finn's family had been known to social services for a number of years. There had been concerns regarding domestic violence and abuse with over 40 police call-outs to the home recorded and being traced back over a number of years and involving Finn's

EXERCISE
- Bearing in mind the methods that Ben engaged with, consider and list:
  — the required principles that underpinned the conversations outlined above
  — the skills required in relation to each of these
  — why it was important for Ben to have the opportunity of engaging with these methods.
- Do you think the conversation with Ben would have been different if these methods were not available? If yes, in what ways?
- What are the main issues emerging from the conversation with Ben?
- Try to write a summary of the main issues for Ben in one or two paragraphs as if you were completing the section of a court report regarding Ben's views and feelings.

mother receiving injuries that required attention from both general practitioners and a local hospital. There were also concerns regarding parental substance misuse (prescription medication and alcohol) that had also resulted in the police being called out to the family home on several occasions. Lastly, both parents experienced some mental health difficulties, especially in terms of suicide threats, requiring intermittent medication and psychiatric input.

The impact of these issues resulted in home conditions being chaotic and unstable for the children. There were occasions when there was no food in the house and when the children were persistently late for school or did not attend at all. Furthermore, the children had been exposed to incidents of violence and disturbed behaviour that unsettled their sleep, their appetites and their concentration at school. Lastly, there were complaints from the neighbours that the children were left to their own devices for long periods of time. The children were eventually removed from the care of their parents when these issues spiralled out of control and it was deemed no longer safe for the children to remain at home. The siblings were separated, with Finn being placed in foster care.

Beginning of conversation and Finn's memories of family life

At the start of the interview, as will be seen below, Finn did not want to talk about anything that I did not already have prior knowledge of. I accepted this boundary using the start of the conversation to confirm that I knew from social services that his father drank. In the early part of my conversation with Finn we confirmed the members of his family and extended family and then the conversation proceeded as follows:

KW: And at the moment you're not living at home with them?
Finn: [*Shakes head. Silence as KW watches Finn pick out a mask from the art materials and then some glitter pens.*]
KW: And can you think of the reasons why you're not living at home with them?
Finn: No.
KW: Shall I tell you some of the reasons that social workers have told me why you can't live at home and you tell me whether they're true or false?
Finn: OK.

KW: OK. The first thing that social workers say is that you can't live at home because daddy used to drink. Is that true or false?

Finn: True.

KW: And what was it like when he used to drink?

Finn: Bad.

KW: Can you remember any of the things that used to go on?

Finn: Yes. [*Time passes as Finn starts to unscrew glitter pen lids and lay out some colours in a row ready to be used to decorate his mask.*]

KW: [*Later in interview*] This is your daddy [*pointing to a coloured pen that Finn has chosen to represent his father*], OK, and sometimes your daddy's drunk, what's he like when he's drunk?

Finn: Falls [*points to the coloured glitter pen he is using, picks it up and it falls over*].

KW: He falls? And if you're, this is, what colour shall I choose for you?

Finn: Green.

KW: Green? This is Finn and he sees his daddy falling over, crash, like that, what does Finn feel like?

Finn: Help him.

KW: [*Later in interview*] Where do you put him if you're trying to lift him up?

Finn: Somewhere warm.

KW: Somewhere warm?

Finn: Shed.

KW: The shed?

Finn: [. . .] Yeah I need red [*beginning to make a mask with the pens that also represent people in his family*].

KW: [*Later in interview*] And what does mummy do?

Finn: Come out.

KW: She comes out? Here she comes. And what, then what happens?

Finn: Where's the green?

KW: Light green? [*Pen passed to Finn.*] So mummy comes to daddy who's outside and what does mummy do then?

Finn: Don't know. Just leaves him out there.

Finn: [*Later in interview*] What's this colour [*making the mask*]?

KW: It's kind of like light orange, that colour is light orange. And then what happened, Finn, if your daddy kept on coming back and back and back?

Finn: Mummy keeps on hitting him. I'm done [*using the completion of his mask as a way of also indicating the end of this part of the conversation*].

KW: You're done. That's lovely.

It can be seen in the excerpt that Finn used the art materials (in this case the pens) symbolically to represent members of his family to talk through some of his memories of life at home. The important skill here was not to judge Finn's choice of method (by responses such as, 'Would it not be better to use these Lego figures?' for example) but to respect and build on Finn's chosen method. Furthermore, it was important not to cast judgement on Finn's experiences by using responses such as, 'that is terrible', but rather to respond in an attentive and empathic manner. Finn also constructed a mask during his conversation with me (see Figure 7.7). Finn was one of the children who did not want to take his work with him and who was comfortable with me using his

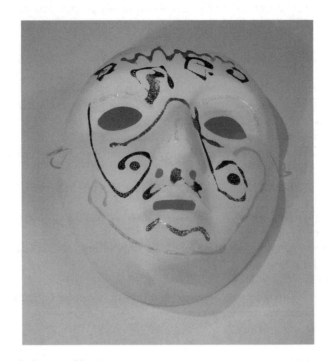

Figure 7.7 A mask decorated by Finn.

work to help social workers improve their practice because, although he felt his social worker did listen to him, he felt they should listen more.

Finn did not indicate in his conversation with me that the mask related to anyone or anything in particular, but he did use it as a vehicle through which he could control the pace and depth of the conversation and by using his concentration on the mask as a way of regulating his eye contact with me.

An example was where Finn used the action of completing the mask to also simultaneously indicate to me that he wished to end the conversation about his father. I responded by respecting this choice and by changing the focus of the conversation by facilitating Finn to reflect on happier memories of life at home. This proved very important to Finn because he had earlier complained that social workers did not believe him when he said he was happy at home whereas he had, in fact, had some good times at home. His mother had also pointed out that the social services assessment of multiple risk factors belied the fact that not all those risks were present all of the time and that their effects were not uniform over time. The following conversation with Finn, which is a continuation from above, indicated this:

KW: And when daddy lived in the house and he wasn't drinking, what was it like then?
Finn: Happy.
KW: Was it? What kind of things did you used to do together that were happy? Can you think of anything?
Finn: Buy my bike.

KW:	Oh yeah. And what colour is your bike?
Finn:	Blue and . . .
KW:	Is there a field at the back of your house, or do you, can you ride it on the roads, are you allowed to ride it on the roads?
Finn:	Well, well, yeah, cos no cars comes up. Want me to show you the way it goes?
KW:	[*KW nods and Finn draws a map with his finger on the table.*]
Finn:	[*Later in interview*] I've got a special bike hat.
KW:	Have you?
Finn:	You can't feel a thing if you, do you want me to show what my hat looks like?
KW:	Yeah, yeah, I'd love you to.
Finn:	This is it [*drawing the shape on the table with his finger*].

Finn's feelings

The conversation around Finn's happy memories, in which he used his fingers to draw as opposed to the methods on offer, led into a further discussion about his feelings as illustrated below:

KW:	Is that one of the things that you miss about home, your bike?
Finn:	Yeah.
KW:	Yeah? And is there anything else you miss about home?
Finn:	Yeah.
KW:	What other things do you miss?
Finn:	Everything!

Part of the reason for Finn's very definitive statement at the end was that following his sudden removal from his family home he had not been allowed to physically revisit it and he missed his local friends, his pet and his belongings. He complained about this in our conversation, knowing that other professionals had been to visit the home when he was no longer there. He did not think this was fair. In Finn's case, as expressed through the methods on offer as well as methods of his own choosing, it was clear that despite what Finn knew of and had experienced in his family, his family life remained very important to him and he still wished to go home, as can be seen below:

KW:	Yeah, you can take that, of course you can. What else makes you happy about home?
Finn:	[*Points to drawing of bike.*]
KW:	Bike?
Finn:	[*Nods.*]
KW:	Things that make you sad?
Finn:	Not going home.
KW:	[*Later in interview*] What would you like to change?
Finn:	Go back to mummy's.
KW:	Go back to mummy's.
Finn:	There's my snake [*referring to a snake he has made out of playdough as he is talking with KW*].

KW: That's nice. It's like mine [*KW has also simultaneously made a snake from playdough*]. Let's say that you go back to mummy's and daddy turns up and the social workers say, 'Oh, you can't go back 'cause it's not safe', what do you think about that?

Finn: Go to my granny's to stay.

KW: OK, so go to granny's?

Finn: To stay with my daddy.

KW: Go back to mummy's, go to granny's to stay with daddy?

Finn: With my daddy comes.

KW: Yes, with my daddy comes, yes, I see.

The conversation with Finn highlights his use of art materials as props and as a vehicle through which he could control the pace, depth and content of the conversation. One issue that could have been further explored was whether Finn had chosen a mask to decorate for any particular reason. During the conversation, as indicated earlier, there was no obvious link between the mask and the content and process of the conversation but that is not to say that there may have been deeper thoughts and feelings that were not accessed during the conversation together. Another interesting point to emerge from the conversation with Finn was, as stated earlier, that he was happy for me to keep the mask. He saw it as connected with our conversation and did not want to take it away with him. Lastly, as said earlier, he was comfortable with the idea that his work could be used to help improve social work practice.

Summary

This chapter has used case studies of conversations with young children to illustrate the use of art materials to explore their understanding, experiences, circumstances, views and feelings. It has been shown how attention to power imbalances, boundaries and ethical issues helped create the right conditions for the conversations to take place.

EXERCISE
- What are the main principles underpinning the conversation with Finn? Where possible, highlight with examples from the excerpts.
- What examples can you find of listening skills, questioning skills and responding skills?
- Give examples of where you think things could have been done differently.
- What are the main issues emerging from the conversation with Finn?
- Write a written summary of Finn's views and feelings as if you are writing a section of a report for a review meeting.
- Think about practical ways that you could ensure that Finn's feelings are properly represented in meetings.

The use of participatory methods, underpinned by the principles reflective of a child rights-based approach in which the choices, individuality and views of young children were respected and valued, brings to life the deeply held views and feelings of young children about their circumstances. The case studies reveal that these young children had memories of their lives at home and of some of the abuse they experienced. Some could also recall their removal from home and the apparent lack of information regarding this. The children experienced a range of feelings since coming into care. For most of them, feelings of self-blame were combined with a strong desire to be reconnected with their families. Lack of space to explore their home lives or the reasons why they had come into care, as well as the lack of opportunity to revisit the places from which they had been suddenly removed or to explore their mixed experiences of alternative state care emerged as a major gap in service provision for these young children. It is within this context that the last chapter makes recommendations for ways forward to address existing gaps in social work practice.

8   Summary and ways forward

Summary of chapter content

The purpose of this chapter is threefold. First, it summarizes the key issues covered in this book regarding the importance of social workers developing meaningful relationships with young children. Specifically, it draws attention to the findings of public inquiries, the value placed on relationships by young children and their social workers and the barriers that currently exist in this crucial area of practice. Second, the chapter outlines the main characteristics of a child rights-based approach, which it argues is necessary to overcome some of the currently identified challenges. The application of a child rights-based approach to real-life case studies of young children between the ages of 4 and 7 years provides the basis from which to explore the principles, methods and skills that enable effective communication with young children. This approach can lead to some commonly held reactions and concerns, which are identified and addressed in detail. Third, the chapter ends by making a series of recommendations as to how social workers and their senior managers can use a child rights-based approach to both fully inform the development of practice guidelines and as an audit tool with the aim of improving their relationships and communication with young children.

Introduction

This book has explored in some detail the ways in which social workers relate to and communicate with young children. Given the current state of social work practice and the influence of the taken-for-granted ways in which social workers view and relate to young children – what has been termed their professional habitus in this book – it is likely that the approaches advocated here will have been challenging to read for some people on at least two levels. First, there is the challenge to people's own beliefs and attitudes. For some, the content of the reported conversations with the children will be shocking. It is quite understandable that some people will have reservations and possibly even objections about creating space for children to talk about such sensitive issues and then placing this work in the public domain. People may also be concerned that allowing children to talk will do more harm than good; that it exposes them to the possibility of exploitation through the misrepresentation of their views; that it falsely raises their expectations; and that, ultimately, it has no long-term benefits. As such there is a need, in this final chapter, to work through some of these issues. Second, and beyond these concerns, for those who accept the approach outlined in this book, there remain many challenges in practice in terms of building relationships and communicating with young children given the organizational context, professional habitus and constraints that exist within the social work profession. Recommendations for ways forward have to both recognize and yet challenge these existing constraints. These too will be explored in detail in this final chapter.

The chapter therefore begins by drawing out the key messages contained in the previous chapters. It starts with those contained in the inquiry reports regarding the failings in social workers' relationships with young children. The book then illustrates how the development of a professional social worker habitus explains many of the similarities in failings identified so consistently through these reports over time. In acknowledging that a key challenge is implementing change at both the organizational and individual levels of the social work profession, the chapter moves on to argue that the UNCRC should be used as the framework onto which broad organizational policy and detailed practice guidelines should be mapped. The application of a child rights-based approach in communicating with young children, drawing attention to the principles, skills and methods used, is then outlined and some of the key messages emerging from this approach identified.

Having summarized the book the chapter then moves on to anticipate and attempt to address some of the common reactions that people may have to a child rights-based approach and to the detailed accounts provided by young children that can emerge through the application of such an approach. These reactions include a fear of causing children harm and exposing them to exploitation, a concern that young children's accounts are not true and/or trustworthy, a worry about how much significance they should attach to what young children say and a query about whether this type of approach can be used with pre-verbal children and children with disabilities. Responses to these worries, concerns and queries are then outlined. The last section of the chapter is concerned with making a series of recommendations to social workers, team managers and those responsible for resource allocation about ways in which they can improve their relationships and communication with young children can be improved.

Summary of the book

Young children and the problems in their relationships with social workers

Young children who come to be known to social services – including those whose accounts are featured in this book – tend to be particularly vulnerable given their family circumstances, their own needs and their care experiences. As noted in Chapter Two, often they come from families with multiple difficulties, including: parental substance dependency; mental/physical ill health; domestic violence; as well as poverty, isolation, poor housing, unemployment and/or single parenthood. They are likely to have experienced some abusive, chaotic, fractured, frightening and/or violent family relationships. Moreover, they often have significant health and educational needs and experience emotional and psychological disturbance. Unfortunately, all of this can be compounded by their experiences when in the care of social services as they undergo multiple placement moves and changes of social worker (Monteith and Cousins 2003; Ward *et al.* 2006; Munro and Ward 2008; Sempik *et al.* 2008; Ward 2009). The facts therefore speak for themselves. These young children are in desperate need of high-quality relationships with their social workers and others caring for them because, as McLeod (2008b: 28) argues, adults having relationships with and 'listening to children can protect children, can enhance their well-being and can lead to improvements in services'.

Despite the particular circumstances of young children known to social services, and their desperate need for consistent and meaningful relationships with adults around them, it was seen in Chapter One that, over the years, inquiry reports into the deaths of young children known to social services have consistently indicated serious failings in this aspect of social work practice with fatal consequences for the children concerned. It was noted that, within the UK, the reports of over 70 child abuse public inquiries have been published since 1945 (Corby *et al.* 1998). As was seen, strikingly similar concerns have repeatedly been raised for over 50 years regarding the quality and nature of social worker relationships with young children. These concerns, set within the context of broader organizational deficits, have included failures by social workers to: visit young children frequently and consistently; see young children alone when visits did take place; engage and communicate with young children directly and personally; complete written records of visits to children; act decisively upon visible cumulative concerns, especially children's weight loss, neglect, bruises and behavioural disturbance; and above all to make the child the focus of the intervention instead of focusing on the parents. These failings are remarkable given their consistency over time, the vulnerabilities of the children concerned and the fact that they have continued to occur despite the emphasis placed on the importance of social workers' relationships with young children in recent reforms to legislation, policy and practice.

The fact that young children known to social services need consistent, positive, safe and meaningful relationships with adults around them has been acknowledged by the government and is now considered a top priority. This is reflected in recent developments in legislation, policies and social work practice, where relationships are seen as crucial in terms of securing young children's well-being, development and rights and in also ensuring effective social work practice at all stages of the social work process, from assessment through to intervention and evaluation (DfES 2006; DCSF 2008a, 2008b, 2009a, 2009b). Perhaps the biggest insight into the importance of relationships, as outlined in Chapter Two, comes from the children themselves. As was seen, research reveals that where children have been able to establish meaningful relationships with their social workers these have been regarded as very important to them (Buchanan *et al.* 1993; Fletcher 1993; Lynes and Goddard 1995; Thomas and O'Kane 1998; Munro 2001; Bell 2002; VCC/NCB 2004; Morgan 2006; NICCY 2006; Leeson 2007; McLeod 2006, 2007, 2008a, 2008b). For these children they valued relationships with their social workers because these mean that someone genuinely takes an interest in them, wants the best for them, enjoys being with them and is also concerned for them (McLeod 2008a, 2008b).

However, despite all that is known about these young children and despite the fact that policy makers and practitioners acknowledge the importance of relationships, failings in social worker relationships with young children persist. In understanding why it is the case that, over many years and in many different places, similar failings in social worker relationships have been identified, Chapter Three has focused on the influence of what has been termed the social work professional habitus. This habitus represents all of those taken-for-granted practices – or habits – that social workers tend to form in response to the routine demands and pressures of the broader organizational context of the social work profession. Elements of the social work professional habitus that have inhibited the building of meaningful relationships with children, described in detail in Chapter Three, include those associated with tasks, trust, threats, theories, training, tools and time.

In terms of *tasks* it was seen that some social workers feel that certain tasks (particularly certain aspects of bureaucratic, assessment and social control tasks) hinder their ability to form meaningful relationships with young children. In particular, the completion of bureaucratic tasks is seen to take priority over spending individual time with children (Le Grand 2007; Gupta and Blewitt 2007; Ruch 2010a, 2010b). Moreover, social control tasks, which might involve undertaking actions that children disagree with, such as removal from family homes, can lead to a situation where children feel unable to *trust* their social workers and avoid having relationships with them (Leeson 2007; McLeod 2007; Winter 2010). Some social workers also tend to avoid relating to young children too closely because they are afraid that this might be a *threat* to children's well-being; causing them more harm than good (Winter 2010). A related issue is that some social workers avoid contact with young children believing that closer contact increases the threat of complaints and false allegations being made (Parton 2006; Green 2007) as well as the threat of aggression and violence from parents (Stanley and Goddard 1997, 2002; Ferguson 2005). Other social workers do not relate to young children as well as they could because of deeply held, often unconscious, beliefs about young children's abilities in which they tend to underestimate their competencies and capacities. These beliefs stem from a narrow and crude interpretation of child development *theories*, which rely on age alone to determine childhood competencies and capacities (Taylor 2004; Holland 2004; Winter 2010).

As argued in Chapter Three, difficulties in building relationships and communicating with young children are further compounded by social workers' lack of access to *training* opportunities, practical *tools* and *time* to engage with young children in a meaningful way. With regard to training, recent reviews (Laming 2009; SWTF 2009a, 2009b) have highlighted the lack of consistency in social work training at degree level with some students not having the opportunity to undertake more specialist courses in communicating with children and also not having placement opportunities to develop relationship and communication skills with young children. Furthermore, once qualified, there remains a lack of access to specialist training courses. In terms of tools there is a lack of resources to purchase and store these and a lack of knowledge and skill as to how to use these effectively (CWDC Research Team 2009 unpublished). These problems are compounded by the lack of time available to build meaningful relationships and communicate with young children (Gupta and Blewitt 2007; Le Grand 2007).

Developing relationships with young children: a child rights-based approach

Chapter Three highlighted that while there are many barriers to social workers developing meaningful relationships with young children there were some important examples of good practice where social workers had built meaningful relationships with children and where opportunities to communicate with them were prioritized. In these situations the work was characterized more by an emphasis on children's rights and children's competencies, which, in turn, created a more appropriate climate for social worker relationships with young children to flourish. Reflecting these themes, and bearing in mind current social work reforms, it was argued in Chapter Four that the United Nations Convention on the Rights of the Child (UNCRC) (UN 1989) should be explicitly and fully adopted as the overarching framework onto which both broad policy and detailed practice guidelines for social work practice with young children should be mapped. This, it was argued, is different from what is currently happening where social work policy and practice guidelines, while making reference to aspects of the UNCRC, do not use the framework in its entirety as the foundation from which to map detailed guidelines.

As explained in Chapter Four, a child rights-based approach means five key things. First, it requires social work practice with young children to be explicitly based upon the four core foundational principles which are at the heart of the UNCRC: the right to non-discrimination (article 2); the best interests principle (article 3); the right to life, survival and development (article 6); and the right to express views freely (article 12). Second, it means that, in all relationships with all children, social workers should have regard for the full range of rights contained in the UNCRC, including their rights to protection from harm, abuse and exploitation, their rights to the provision of services including health, education and social security, and their rights to participation in decision-making, and cultural and leisure activities. Third, it means that social workers should have regard for the detailed interpretation of specific articles as laid out in the various General Comments produced by the UN Committee and that they should fully engage with the implications of these for their own individual and organizational practice with young children. Fourth, it means that in all relationships with children, their rights should be seen as indivisible and interdependent so that children's rights have to be seen as a whole, such that the realization of any particular right is dependent on the realization of the others. Finally, it means understanding that paying attention to these principles and rights is not an optional extra but a legal requirement.

Given the above, it was argued that social workers are, therefore, required to conduct their relationships with young children differently. For example, in determining a child's best interests (article 3) they are required to ascertain the views of the child (article 12). In so doing they are required to start from the assumption that the child, regardless of their age, can engage in a meaningful relationship (article 2 UNCRC; UN 2005, 2007, 2009) and can express their views (articles 2, 5, 12–14 UNCRC; UN 2005, 2007, 2009). This in turn is dependent on the provision of appropriate, accessible information and guidance by the social worker to the child concerned (articles 5, 13, 17 UNCRC) in line with children's evolving capacities (article 5 UNCRC; UN 2009).

It was also argued in Chapter Four that what a child rights-based approach also requires is that all social work processes with children (which include assessment, planning, decision-making, implementation of plans and the review/evaluation of plans) should be transparent and informative, voluntary, respectful, relevant, child-friendly, inclusive, supported by training, safe and sensitive to risk and accountable (UN 2009: 26–7). What these principles mean in practice is that all children should have access to appropriately pitched information that reflects the child's competencies and capacities so that the reasons and purpose of social work involvement is clear and transparent. Furthermore, it means that children should not feel coerced or pressurized into engaging in any part of the social work process but rather it should be with their consent and voluntary. Moreover, it means that social workers should be respectful of the individuality, choices, freedoms and views of the child in their relationships with young children. Also, the methods and skills they use should not alienate and further marginalize young children but be inclusive and child-friendly, reflecting young children's skills, interests and capacities.

Importantly too, as was also stressed in Chapter Four, social workers should ensure that they pay attention to the safety of the child when seeking their views. This means accepting that in certain situations there may be a risk to children by seeking their views (for example, in situations with known familial violence) and thus recognizing the need to develop ways of addressing and managing that risk (UN 2009). It also means paying attention to power imbalances in the social worker–child relationship and addressing these by, for example, avoiding the use of jargon. Attention to boundaries is also an important aspect in creating a safe atmosphere for children. In particular, social workers should be clear about their own role and the limits to their own expertise. Where necessary they should call on the help of trained therapists to deal with the deeply held and unresolved feelings that young children might harbour and that might have a detrimental impact on their well-being in the short and long term. Finally, it was stressed that all work involving children should be accountable to the children concerned (UN 2009). What this means in practice is that children should be involved in decision-making and they should be told about how and in what ways their own views had an impact on the decisions made.

Relationships with young children: a child rights-based approach in action

Having outlined the principles of a child rights-based approach, Chapters Five, Six and Seven then moved on to provide case studies involving real-life conversations with young children to illustrate a child rights-based approach in action. Chapter Five detailed the stages and skills of the communication process. The chapter showed the skills required in establishing rapport with young children and then provided illustrations of ways to question, listen and respond that respected the individuality, choices and freedoms of young children and that also paid attention to power imbalances, boundaries and ethical issues (Trevithick 2005; Koprowska 2008; Lefevre 2008; McLeod 2008a, 2008b; UN 2009). Crucially what Chapter Five did was to show that conversations were structured around engaging with young children to establish answers to questions such as, 'What does the world look like through your eyes?' 'What is it like to be in your shoes for a day?' and 'How best can I help you connect with me to share with me what your experiences and feelings are?' While these changes might appear subtle, it was explained that they reflect a more fundamental shift in thinking about the value and importance we attach to children and our relationships with them and how we go about communicating with young children in practice.

Chapter Six then focused on the use of participatory methods with young children to gain their views. While this chapter acknowledged that the range of methods is limitless (Crompton 1980; Koprowska 2008; McLeod 2008b; Lefevre 2008, 2010; SCIE 2010), it attempted to illustrate some of these by focusing on the methods used in the current research. These included the use of reality boxes that comprised shoeboxes which young children decorated to depict an external image of themselves on the outside of the box (what they thought they looked like to the outside world) and an internal image of themselves inside the box (what their real thoughts and feelings were). Other methods included the use of props (including an unplugged telephone and old computer) and the use of arts and crafts.

Chapter Six then illustrated the application of a child rights-based approach to the use of such methods, which, it was argued comprised four key principles. First, attention was paid to ethical issues including securing consent to engage in a conversation with a child, being clear about the limits to confidentiality and ensuring the provision of accessible, relevant information about the purpose of conversations and what will happen to the information gained. Second, attention was paid to power imbalances in the adult–child relationship with the aim of consciously reducing their negative impact wherever possible by the social worker paying attention to their facial expressions, tone of voice and body language, for example. Third, attention was paid to boundaries by being clear with a child about the limits to the social worker role and their expertise and thus referring the child to more specialist services where necessary/appropriate. Fourth, and finally, respect for the worth and value of each child was shown through respect for their individuality, their competencies and capacities, their choices and freedoms and the views they express.

Chapter Seven illustrated all of the above principles, skills and methods in action though real-life detailed case studies involving in-depth conversations with young children between the ages of 4 and 7 years old. The chapter revealed that, within the context of a child rights-based approach, young children were capable of engaging in detailed conversations regarding their experiences, perspectives and feelings. These detailed accounts of young children are some of the first of their kind to be placed in the public domain and, as such, it was explained in Chapter Seven how attention to ethical issues has been a priority in this research process in terms of seeking the consent of the children and being clear about anonymity and the limits to confidentiality. Some of the young children described how they had lived with risk and harm within their family homes before social workers intervened, variously describing memories of being locked in bedrooms, hungry, frightened and of witnessing violence and substance misuse.

They also recounted their experiences of removal from their family homes, which had often come as a complete shock and without warning, preparation and/or information. Since living in state care the young children described some positive feelings regarding new relationships with new carers but also a range of more negative and unresolved feelings around loss, sadness and anger. Significantly some of the children spoke of feelings that appeared to amount to self-blame, believing that it was their own actions towards their parents, rather than vice versa, which led them to be in care. Furthermore, although some of the young children had been living away from home for a long time their family members were still very significant. The young children's unresolved feelings appeared to be compounded by the lack of access to information and the lack of opportunity, in their relationships with social workers and others, to explore their circumstances and to come to terms with their pasts.

Chapter Seven also argued that while care needs to be taken not to generalize from this handful of conversations they do very powerfully illustrate how young children can engage in meaningful conversations about their perspectives within the context of relationships, and that to deny them the chance of developing these relationships and sharing their perspectives can cause long-term damage to their emotional and psychological well-being.

Common reactions to young children's perspectives

As mentioned in the introduction to this chapter, given the nature of the conversations recounted and the existing perceptions of young children and beliefs about their development and capabilities, there are likely to be many responses to the arguments set out in this book and as summarized above. Some are likely to question the relevance of the work and how much can be read into what the children say, whereas others will be more explicitly rejecting of the whole approach. In this section some of the most likely reactions are anticipated and outlined, and responses to these are provided.

'This type of work causes more harm than good.'

For some people, there will be a very real concern that by encouraging children to revisit and reflect upon their experiences we may actually be risking them becoming re-traumatized. As such, it could well be argued that some things are best left where they belong – in the past. While these concerns are understandable, it is important to be aware of the difference between a child becoming upset when talking about sensitive issues and becoming re-traumatized. Part of coming to terms with what has happened necessarily involves reconnecting with the emotions that those past events evoked. Moreover, unless such emotions are addressed they are unlikely simply to go away and children will, periodically, return to them of their own volition and thus suffer the negative effects of doing so without ever being given the support and skills required to work them through. It is for this reason that it is important to give children the opportunity to explore and express these emotions so that they can be acknowledged and understood safely within the context of supportive relationships. All the children in this book had supportive relationships with their carers. Having said this, it is also important to ensure that other appropriate support mechanisms are in place prior to conversations beginning and this should, as was made available in the current research, include the input of a trained therapist with an expertise in working with young children.

With regard to the young children who featured in this book, clear protocols were established and put in place before the first conversations took place. Where young children discussed harm (past or present) these details were passed on to the social workers who were still involved in the lives of the children, reflecting the fact that social services had acquired legal parental responsibility for the children through the courts. If children became upset then a named person known to the child could be called on to offer the child support once their conversations with me had ended, even if their feelings did not merge until a few days later. In my work there was no occasion where this was needed. In fact carers of the children reported that the young children appeared very positive about the conversations and that in the case of Aine, whose conversations were reported at length in Chapter Five, she was reported subsequently as appearing relieved.

It is worth also noting that all of the children involved in the research embraced the opportunity to talk at the time the conversations were taking place and some did not want those conversations to end. Social workers were informed of these reactions and it was suggested that the children might benefit from further conversations of a similar nature. Within this context, and where children did begin to talk about their negative memories, it would actually have been inappropriate to stop these conversations as this could have left the child with the impression that what they were saying was wrong or not valued. Rather, it was imperative to handle their conversations with respect and sensitivity. It is this type of response that social workers should be seeking to develop with young children.

'This type of work can lead to the perspectives of vulnerable children being misrepresented.'

It is possible for social workers to form fixed views about what they think is in a child's best interests before they even speak with the child concerned. With this in mind it is possible that, when they communicate with young children, they might unintentionally and subconsciously only hear what they want to hear. By the same subtle processes they might also accord more significance to those views that concur with their own and/or that support a proposed plan and they might thus emphasize certain aspects of the child's views in reports and meetings and exclude those that they disagree with. They might also try and provide a coherent account when, in fact, the expressed views of the child are conflicting and ambiguous. The potential for these types of misrepresentation is greater given the status of the young children and because of age-related discrimination and the tendency of some social workers to underestimate their capacities.

In response there are practical measures that can and should be used to help address the potential for misrepresentation, as outlined in Chapter Six. First, social workers need to provide methods and tools for conversations with children that allow children to reflect on their views and that are non-directional; that is, not designed to elicit a certain response. Second, social workers need to acknowledge exactly what their own views are and how these might differ from or concur with the views expressed by the child. As part of this, social workers should accurately present the entirety of a conversation with a child rather than an edited or refined version that supports the social worker's own decision, assessment or preferred course of action. Third, where possible, children should be actively involved in helping to decide how and through which medium their views will be shared. This would help those who believe that young children's views have been misconstrued or that they are being exploited in any way.

'Children's views are not reliable and cannot be trusted.'

Often people will react, subconsciously if not consciously, to young children's views with queries about their reliability and trustworthiness. These reactions include doubts about young children's recall abilities, as well as concerns that young children may feel pressurized into sharing only certain views and/or saying what they think another person wants to hear. This, in turn, leads to the reliability of children's views being questioned, especially if they vary slightly, and are not replicated faithfully, over time or in different contexts.

There is a great deal of psychological and social research regarding young children's recall abilities and with varied findings on this question. While there is not space to provide a detailed overview of the knowledge base required to address the points in detail it is important for social workers to be familiar with the general findings of this research which suggests that young children can recall reliable information so long as interviewers engage appropriately in conversation with them and adapt their style and methods to suit the individual needs of the child (Dockett and Perry 2007; Larsson and Lamb 2009).

The reliability or trustworthiness of a child's account may be compromised if young children feel awkward or uncomfortable and/or are pressurized into saying what they think others want to hear. This reflects a broader concern about young children's suggestibility (i.e. their acceptance of and acting upon the suggestions of others) and/or a concern that they may have been coached. With this in mind, it is important for social workers to pay attention to the contexts of conversations. As stated in Chapter Five, clarity of purpose, attention to the location, structure and content of the conversation and a focus on the methods should help reduce any pressure that the child might feel under.

Lastly, some people query the reliability and trustworthiness of young children's accounts because the children might have modified the perspectives they express to different people at different times. Given that all conversation is a social process that is context- and time-specific, it is impossible for anyone (not just children) to replicate in its entirety a previous conversation. It is much more likely that different aspects will be emphasized to different people at different times, in different contexts and that additional information, hitherto unexpressed and hidden, may also come into the consciousness. Rather than seeing this as indicative of unreliability, this should be accepted as a natural part of the conversational process that is common to all human beings rather than specific to just children.

> 'Given their limited understanding we shouldn't place much weight on the young child's views in any case.'

The question of what weight should be attached to a child's views relates to how much influence a child's views should have in determining a decision, an outcome or a course of action. It is important to note that competence can be experientially related as opposed to simply age-related. This fact has to be taken into account in making a determination about the weight to be attached to the child's view. Furthermore, in determining that weight the UN Committee in General Comment No. 12 (UN 2009: 7) states that 'it is not necessary that the child has comprehensive knowledge of all aspects of the matter [. . .] but that she or he has sufficient understanding to be capable of appropriately forming his or her own views on the matter'. As can be seen these points illustrate that, far from simply ruling out a child's view on the basis of their age, young children's views should be given weight in decision-making processes. One practical way of doing this, as I have observed in court proceedings, is to start with the child's expressed views and then to ask the question whether these are in their best interests and, if not, why not.

> 'It is not possible to use the approach outlined in this book with pre-verbal children.'

For some there is a belief that very young children who are pre-verbal cannot express their views or feelings and thus that it is not possible to communicate with them using a child rights-based approach. However, babies are social beings and anyone who has direct experience of caring for a baby will know that long before they have the words, they are able to communicate very powerfully through a whole host of ways including movements, smiles, giggles, cries, gazes, gurgles, facial movements, agitation and excitement. Moreover, most parents are able to tell the difference between different types of crying. Babies seek out comfort from others by responding positively to their warmth and becoming distressed if others are distressed (Alderson *et al.* 2006). It is not long before they start pointing to people and objects, start to recognize words and to form their own. In this respect, very young children's capacities are recognized by the UN Committee (UN 2005: 7, para. 14) that states:

> Young children are acutely sensitive to their surroundings and very rapidly acquire understanding of the people, places and routines in their lives, along with awareness of their own unique identity. They make choices and communicate their feelings, ideas and wishes in numerous ways, long before they are able to communicate through the conventions of spoken or written language.

Furthermore, as illustrated by Alderson *et al.* (2006), a child rights-based approach is applicable even to newborn babies. Communication with pre-verbal children is, therefore, not only possible but is an essential part of a social worker's role. However, it does rely upon the development of highly attuned observation skills that are both informed by and help inform an understanding of the child's development, personality, temperament and relationships within their social context (Turney 2008; Lefevre 2010). The best way of acquiring these observation skills is, as argued in Chapter Four, through regular contact with babies and very small children such as in day care and nursery settings. In acquiring these observational skills social workers need to learn ways of presenting their observations that reflect the individuality of each child rather than simply trying to fit their observations into checklists that, while providing helpful guidelines, do not capture the individuality of each very young child.

> 'The approach outlined in this book is also not appropriate for young children with disabilities.'

For some people, there is also a belief that it is not possible to communicate with young children with learning, visual or hearing disabilities and that these children are not capable of expressing their views. This reaction stems from a deficit view of the competencies and capacities of children with these types of disabilities to relate to others and to communicate their views. However, the UNCRC recognizes and challenges this deficit view. Children with disabilities are mentioned as a particular group of children requiring special attention in terms of the right to 'enjoy a full and decent life, in conditions which ensure dignity, promote self-reliance and facilitate the child's active participation in the community' (article 23 UNCRC, UN 1989).

Furthermore, the UN Committee has published a General Comment (UN 2007) regarding the rights of children with disabilities in recognition of the discrimination and exclusion they experience because of the attitudes and practices of people around them. In particular, General Comment No. 7 (UN 2007: 3, para. 8) states:

> Discrimination takes place – often de facto – in various aspects of the life and development of children with disabilities. As an example, social discrimination and stigmatization leads to their marginalization and exclusion, and may even threaten their survival and development if it goes as far as physical or mental violence against children with disabilities. Discrimination in service provision excludes them from education and denies them access to quality health and social services [. . .] Social stigma, fears, overprotection, negative attitudes, misbeliefs and prevailing prejudices against children with disabilities remain strong in many communities and lead to the marginalization and alienation of children with disabilities.

Social workers' communication with children with disabilities should, therefore, be premised on knowledge, skills and values that challenge rather than collude with discrimination and exclusion; it is simply not acceptable to avoid forming relationships and communicating with young children with disabilities on the basis of the misconception that it cannot be done or that there is a lack of knowledge as to how it should be done. It is possible to form relationships and communicate with young children with disabilities and there are a myriad of ways in which any child, whatever their disability, is able to express their feelings and views (Lefevre 2008; Marchant 2008; Koprowska 2008).

> 'This is all well and good in theory but in practice I just don't have the time to do this, given the size of my caseload.'

A final concern likely to be raised by some is that forming relationships and communicating with young children is great in principle but impossible to achieve in practice given the lack of time. However, in response to this point it is simply worth noting that had anyone spent time developing a meaningful relationship and communicating with the children in the inquiries reported in Chapter One then it is likely that the horror they were enduring would have come to light much earlier and that they would probably still be alive, given that social workers involved would have stepped in to remove those children from those circumstances. Indeed, this was the very conclusion reached by Crompton in relation to Maria Colwell when she stated that the tragedy 'might have been averted if someone had paid proper attention and endeavoured to communicate directly with [her]' (Crompton 1980: 7). Furthermore, for those young children struggling to make sense of who they are and where they have come from, the availability of a meaningful relationship with a social worker can make all the difference. The point of all of this, therefore, is to remind social workers that, through improved relationships and more effective communication, children can be better protected and their emotional and psychological well-being enhanced and that, ultimately, a child rights-based approach is a legal requirement, not a luxury optional extra.

Moving forward

With all of these points in mind, it is important to conclude the book with some practical recommendations for future practice. At the outset it is important to recognize the organizational constraints that the social work profession works within and to acknowledge that the profession is currently underfunded and that there is thus a responsibility on the government to appropriately fund child protection work. Social workers who work with children and families are clearly under-resourced, with too many social workers carrying caseloads that are too high and too many social workers really struggling to find any time to develop meaningful relationships with any of the children on their caseloads. Unless the issue of resourcing is fully addressed, it will be impossible for individual social workers and their team managers to fully change the way they operate. However, while acknowledging this fundamental point, the focus of this book has been more limited in nature with respect to the social work profession itself and with how social workers' might develop better and more effective relationships with young children. As such, the discussion that follows reflects this more limited focus and provides recommendations specifically for individual social workers, their team managers and also those responsible for service planning and resource allocation.

Recommendations for social workers

1. Use the UNCRC as a guide for daily practice and as an audit tool

The UNCRC is a comprehensive document that covers most aspects of children's lives and provides detailed guidance on how social workers should conduct their relationships with young children. As has been shown, the UNCRC tells social workers that they have a duty to respect and uphold children's rights to: protection from harm, abuse, exploitation and discrimination (articles 2, 19, 20–23, 32–38); provision of services in education, health, social security, leisure, play and emotional well-being (articles 23–28, 30, 31, 39, 40); and participation in terms of expressing views freely, having those views taken into account in decision-making and of participation in cultural, artistic, recreational and leisure activities (articles 12–15, 30, 31).

There is also no lower age limit to these rights and there are no conditions attached to these rights being conferred. being conferred. Social workers therefore cannot 'cherry pick' which rights they choose to focus on. As explained in previous chapters, all rights are regarded as inter-dependent and indivisible in that the implementation of any particular right depends on the implementation of others. Because of this it is important that social workers read carefully and become fully acquainted with the provisions contained in the UNCRC and that they should also use it as an audit tool to examine daily practice and to highlight what rights are being upheld and what rights are being breached. Moreover, information on breaches should be collated by social workers and passed on to team managers.

2. Begin with the best interests of the child

Under the UNCRC a primary consideration in all work with children is the principle of identifying and upholding their best interests (article 3). The young child is, therefore, the primary focus of a social worker's involvement in a family. It is not the parents who are the primary focus or other family members, and neither are other professionals the primary focus. While these may all seek to exert undue influence, the key issue is that it is the child him/herself and their best interests that should be the social worker's primary concern. It is, therefore, important that social workers see each child as an individual in their own right of worth and dignity (preamble) and accept that they may well have wishes and feelings that may differ from the views of their parents or other adults involved in their lives. As such, it is essential that social workers relate directly to the young child, and ascertain their experiences and perspectives, as part of the process of determining what is in their best interests.

3. Develop a direct and meaningful relationship with the child

Given the above it is therefore important that social workers develop a direct and mean-ingful relationship with every young child. Social workers have a duty to ensure that every child has the opportunity to express their views freely on all decisions affecting them (article 12 UNCRC, UN 2009: 15, paras 70–4). It is therefore their *individual responsibility* and *duty* to establish a personal relationship with every young child based on individual face-to-face communication. Other professionals must not be relied upon to do what is their own individual duty and responsibility.

In building a relationship with a young child, social workers have to begin with the assumption that young children are capable of expressing their views (UN 2009: 6, para. 20). There is no age limit on the expression of views (UN 2009: 6, para. 21) and it is not up to the child to first prove their capacity (UN 2009: 6, para. 20). Furthermore, in building relationships and communicating with children, social workers have to create opportunities for every young child to express their views by the provision of information (article 13), space, time, and suitable methods and in the most appropriate environment (UN 2009: 26–7, para. 134). Lastly, social workers are required to respect the individuality of each child and their competencies, capacities and choices, even when their views are at variance with your own.

4. Represent children's views fully, fairly and accurately

In all meetings, court hearings and reports young children's views should be fully, fairly and accurately represented. Social workers must avoid emphasizing or minimizing a child's own views to support their own line of thinking. In order to ensure that representation is as accurate as possible social workers must involve the child as much as possible in sharing their views in a meeting or decision-making forum by, for example, collaborating with the child to choose the format, the order, the words and/or the work that illustrates their views (article 13 UNCRC, UN 2009: 26–7, para. 134). Lastly, in terms of accountability, social workers have a duty to inform the child of the outcome of any decisions made, how their views have been interpreted and what influence their views had on any decisions made (UN 2009: 26–7, para. 134).

5. Monitor own practice and report problems to your line manager

Finally, it is important that social workers use the UNCRC as an audit tool to keep a note of any barriers that are encountered in building relationships and communicating with young children, whether these stem from their own personal reactions or lack of skills or, alternatively, from parental resistance or from organizational issues such as resources, tools, training and time. It is important that any such barriers are noted and raised by the social worker in supervision meetings with their line manager and that such meetings are used to discuss and agree specific ways to address these, which the social worker must then keep a note of. Examples include the fact that, if faced with a series of competing caseload demands, one of the social worker's priorities should be her/his relationships with young children. Social workers should keep a note of all the other tasks they have been unable to complete which should then be passed on to your team manager. This list could also be used in supervision to identify what is expected in terms of training and support to build relationships and communicate with young children. These could be indicated in the social worker's personal training development plan and followed through. It is recognized, as indicated by Simmonds (2010), that this will only be possible within the context of a supportive, well-functioning supervision relationship. Part of the social worker's responsibility may therefore include drawing out those aspects of the supervision relationship that hinder the development of relationships with children.

Recommendations for team managers

1. Ensure the team's familiarity with the UNCRC and the UN General Comments

Team managers have a duty and a responsibility to ensure that they, and their team, are fully aware of the UNCRC and the UN General Comments. This could be achieved through information-sharing sessions within team meetings, or by bringing in outside speakers and/or by the development of audit tools within the team, for example.

2. Refocus the process of supervision to take account of the quality (rather than the quantity) of social worker relationships with young children

Part of the process of supervision should include a focus on the quality of social worker relationships with the young children known to them. Assessments of the quality of the social worker relationship could include seeking answers in supervision to indicators such as: when and how communication with the young child took place, what issues were discussed using what methods, what information emerged, what feelings and emotional responses were evoked, what observations were made, what records have been kept, what barriers exist in further developing the relationship with the child and what can be done to address those barriers. Furthermore, in case files, reports and meetings do not accept practice that states that the child was too young to express a view. Rather, be clear that all children can express a view and that social workers need to demonstrate how and by what methods, principles and skills they have tried to establish these views.

3. Monitor and keep a note of barriers that are identified as affecting the ability of social workers to develop relationships with children and use the data to advocate for change

The UNCRC should be used as a framework for monitoring daily social worker practice with young children. Where the individual, personal and direct relationship between a social worker and a child is likely to be compromised because of the imposition of other duties, the relationship should be the priority. A note should be kept of other tasks that have not been completed as a result of this aspect of work being prioritized. This information should then be passed on to those responsible for resource allocation to illustrate the impact on daily social worker practice of prioritizing the relational aspects of work with young children. This process is much more in keeping with the active defence of children's rights rather than the silent acceptance of practice that falls short of the mark given the organizational constraints within which social workers have to operate. These recommendations do suggest the need for a more relationship-based style of management and leadership that, as indicated by Turney *et al.* (2010), manages to combine the functions of governance and accountability as well as support and advocacy.

Recommendations to those responsible for service planning and resource allocation

1. Use the UNCRC as the framework for mapping on broad policy statements and detailed practice guidelines for social workers working with children

The UNCRC should be used as the starting point for the development of policies and practices regarding young children known to social services. It should be used as the basis to develop training programmes, forms for meetings, case file records, court reports and to develop audit tools for use by managers and social workers. It is, thus, important that time is spent, if it has not been done already, in conducting a strategic review of existing services and not only assessing them against the standards contained in the UNCRC but also identifying and developing procedures, as well as commissioning additional services as appropriate in order to ensure that these standards are met.

2. Develop a strategy regarding indicators of quality in social worker relationships with young children that, where possible, involve children in their development

As part of the wider strategic review of existing services and the development of processes aimed at monitoring such services and practices and ensuring compliance with the UNCRC is the need to focus specifically on the quality of social worker relationships with young children. This issue of the quality of social worker–child relationships is a crucial component missing in all of the bureaucratic tasks that accompany the social work role. This requires urgent attention. Indicators of what is meant by a quality relationship and how that could be denoted should be developed with the input of young children. These indicators could be integrated into the forms currently used in review meetings for children in care, into current case file record formats and into the existing court report formats. This would lead to more accountability within the profession concerning the quality of their direct, personal relationships with children and make it more of a priority than it is now.

Conclusion

This book has been about social worker relationships with young children, the importance of those relationships, the barriers that exist and the use of a child rights-based approach to successfully dismantle those barriers and to build meaningful and effective relationships with young children. There is no denying the fact that achieving this is a tall order. As stated in General Comment No. 12 regarding the right of children to be heard,

> [a]chieving meaningful opportunities for the implementation of article 12 will necessitate dismantling the legal, political, economic, social and cultural barriers that currently impede children's opportunity to be heard and their access to participation in all matters affecting them. It requires a preparedness to challenge assumptions about children's capacities, and to encourage the development of environments in which children can build and demonstrate capacities. It also requires a commitment to resources and training.
>
> (UN 2009: 28, para. 135)

However, it cannot be emphasized enough just how important meaningful and effective social worker relationships with young children are, even if it is a tall order. Ultimately, of course, relationships are about protecting children and safeguarding them from harm. We need to look no further than the horrors that have been revealed in successive child abuse inquiries to understand this fact. However, relationships are also about ensuring young children's rights to effective provision and participation. All these are indivisible – their protection depends upon their provision and participation. This child rights-based framework requires a change in the way that social workers think about young children, the way that they practise and the ways in which they are supported by their employers. It is hoped that this book offers an important contribution to that journey of change.

Bibliography

A National Voice (ANV) (2007) *Care Matters: A National Voice Response*, London: A National Voice.

Adcock, M., White, R. and Rowlands, O. (1983) *The Administrative Parent: A Study of the Assumption of Parental Rights and Duties*, London: British Agencies for Adoption and Fostering.

Adoption and Children Act (2002) Available online: www.opsi.gov.uk/acts/acts2002/ukpga_20020038_en_1

Alderson, P. (1993) *Children's Consent to Surgery*, Buckingham: Open University Press.

—— (2000) 'Convention on the rights of the child: some common criticisms and suggested responses', *Child Abuse Review*, 9, 439–43.

—— (2000/2008) *Young Children's Rights: Exploring Beliefs, Principles and Practice*, London: Jessica Kingsley Publishers.

Alderson, P., Killen, M. and Hawthorne, J. (2006) 'The participation rights of premature babies', *International Journal of Children's Rights*, 13, 31–50.

Alderson, P. and Morrow, V. (2010) *Ethics, Social Research and Consulting With Children and Young People*, London: Sage.

Aldgate, J., Rose, W. and Jeffery, C. (2006) *The Developing World of the Child*, London: Jessica Kingsley Publishers.

Aldgate, J. and Seden, J. (2006) 'Direct work with children' in J. Aldgate, W. Rose and C. Jeffery (eds) *The Developing World of the Child*, London: Jessica Kingsley Publishers.

Anderson, D. (2000) 'Coping strategies and burnout among veteran child protection workers', *Child Abuse and Neglect*, 24(6), 839–48.

Asquith, S., Clark, C. and Waterhouse, L. (2005) *The Role of the Social Worker in the 21st Century: A Literature Review*, Edinburgh: Scottish Executive.

Backett-Milburn, K. and McKie, L. (1999) 'A critical appraisal of the draw and write technique', *Health Education Research: Theory and Practice*, 14(3), 387–98.

Baldry, S. and Kemmis, J. (1998) 'What is it like to be looked after by a local authority?', *British Journal of Social Work*, 28(4), 129–36.

Bannister, A., Barrett, K. and Shearer, E. (eds) (1997) *Listening to Children: The Professional Response to Hearing the Abused Child*, Chichester: John Wiley & Sons.

Barker, J. and Weller, S. (2003) '"Is it fun?" Developing children centred research methods', *International Journal of Sociology and Social Policy*, 23(1), 33–58.

Bebbington, A. C. and Miles, J. B. (1989) 'The background of children who enter local authority care', *British Journal of Social Work*, 19, 349–68.

Bell, M. (2002) 'Promoting children's rights through the use of relationship', *Child and Family Social Work*, 7, 1–11.

Blewitt, J., Lewis, J. and Tunstill, J. (2007) *The Changing Roles and Tasks of Social Work: A Literature Informed Discussion Paper*, London: General Social Care Council.

Blom-Cooper, L. (1985) *A Child in Trust: The Report of the Panel of Inquiry into the Circumstances Surrounding the Death of Jasmine Beckford*, London: London Borough of Brent.

—— (1987) *A Child in Mind: The Report of the Commission of Inquiry into the Circumstances Surrounding the Death of Kimberley Carlisle*, London: London Borough of Greenwich.

Bogues, S. (2008) *People Work Not Just Paperwork: What People Told Us during the Consultation Conducted for the NISCC Roles and Tasks of Social Work Project*, Belfast: Northern Ireland Social Care Council.

Bourdieu, P. (1972) *Outline of a Theory of Practice*, Cambridge: Cambridge University Press.

—— (1999) 'Understanding' in P. Bourdieu *et al.* (eds) *The Weight of the World: Social Suffering in Contemporary Society*, Cambridge: Polity Press.

Bourdieu *et al.* (1999) *The Weight of the World: Social Suffering in Contemporary Society*, Cambridge: Polity Press.

Brandon, M., Bailey, S., Belderson, P., Gardner, R., Sidebotham, P., Dodsworth, J., Warren, C. and Black, J. (2009) *Understanding Serious Case Reviews and their Impact: A Biennial Analysis of Serious Case Reviews 2005–07*, London: Department for Children, Schools and Families.

Buchanan, A., Wheal, A., Walder, D., Macdonald, S. and Coker, R. (1993) *Dolphin Project: Answering Back; Report by Young People being Looked After on the Children Act 1989*, Southampton: Centre for Evaluative and Developmental Research, University of Southampton.

Bushin, N. (2007) 'Interviewing children in their homes: developing flexible techniques and putting ethical principles into practice', *Children's Geographies*, 5(3), 235–51.

Butler-Sloss, Lord Justice E. (1988) *Report of the Inquiry into Child Abuse in Cleveland 1987*, Cmd 412, London: HMSO.

Care Matters (2006) *Transforming the Lives of Children and Young People in Care*, Cmd 6932, London: Department for Education and Skills.

—— (2007) *Consultation Responses*, London: Department for Education and Skills.

—— (2008) *Time to Deliver for Children in Care: An Implementation Plan*, London: Department for Children, Schools and Families.

Childcare Act (2006) Available online: www.opsi.gov.uk/acts/acts2006/pdf/ukpga_20060021_en.pdf

Childhoods 2005 Oslo (2005) Conference website, Available online: http://childhoods2005.uio.no/

Children Act (1975) Available online: www.opsi.gov.uk/acts/acts1975/pdf/ukpga_19750072_en.pdf

—— (1989) Available online: www.opsi.gov.uk/acts/acts1989/ukpga_19890041_en_1

—— (2004) Available online: www.opsi.gov.uk/Acts/acts2004/ukpga_20040031_en_1

Children and Young Persons Act (2008) Available online: www.opsi.gov.uk/acts/acts2008/pdf/ukpga_20080023_en.pdf

Children and Young People's Unit (CYPU) (2001) *Learning to Listen: Core Principles for the Involvement of Children and Young People*, London: Children and Young Persons Unit.

Children (Leaving Care) Act (2000) Available online: www.opsi.gov.uk/acts/acts2000/ukpga_20000035_en_1

Children (Scotland) Act (1995) Available online: www.opsi.gov.uk/ACTS/acts1995/ukpga_19950036_en_1

Children (Northern Ireland) Order, The (1995) Available online: www.opsi.gov.uk/si/si1995/uksi_19950755_en_1

Children's Legal Centre (CLC) (1984) *It's My Life Not Theirs*, London: Children's Legal Centre.

Children's Rights Alliance for England (CRAE) (2009) *Beyond Article 12: The Local Implementation of the UN Convention on the Rights of the Child in England*, London: Children's Rights Alliance for England.

Children's Workforce Development Council (CWDC) (2009) *Early Identification, Assessment of Needs and Intervention: The Common Assessment Framework for Children and Young People*, Leeds: Children's Workforce Development Council.

—— (2010) *Refreshing the Common Core of Skills and Knowledge*, Leeds: Children's Workforce Development Council.

Children's Workforce Development Council (CWDC) Research Team (2009) 'Newly qualified social workers: a report on consultations with newly qualified social workers, employers and those in higher education', unpublished.

Christensen, P. (2004) 'Children's participation in ethnographic research: issues of power and representation', *Children and Society*, 18, 165–76.

Christensen, P. and James, A. (eds) (2008a) *Research with Children: Perspectives and Practices* (2nd edn), London: Routledge.

—— (2008b) 'Researching children and childhood: cultures of communication' in P. Christensen and A. James (eds) *Research with Children: Perspectives and Practices* (2nd edn), London: Routledge.

Clark, A. and Moss, P. (2001) *Listening to Young Children: The Mosaic Approach*, London: National Children's Bureau.

Clark, A. and Statham, J. (2005) 'Listening to young children: experts in their own lives', *Adoption and Fostering*, 29(1), 45–56.

Cleaver, H., Cawson, P., Gorin, S. and Waller, S. (eds) (2009) *Safeguarding Children: A Shared Responsibility*, Chichester: Wiley-Blackwell.

Cleaver, H., Unell, I. and Aldgate, J. (1999) *Children's Needs – Parenting Capacity: The impact of Parental Mental Illness, Problem Alcohol and Drug Use, and Domestic Violence on Children's Development*, London: The Stationery Office.

Cleaver, H., Walker, S. and Meadows, P. (2004) *Assessing Children's Needs and Circumstances: The Impact of the Assessment Framework*, London: Jessica Kingsley Publishers.

Cleaver, H., Walker, S., Scott, J., Cleaver, D., Rose, W., Ward, H. and Pithouse, A. (2008) *The Integrated Children's System: Enhancing Social Work and Inter-Agency Practice*, London: Jessica Kingsley Publishers.

Coates, E. and Coates, A. (2006) 'Young children talking and drawing', *International Journal of Early Years Education*, 14(3), 221–41.

Connolly, P. (2008) 'Race, gender and critical reflexivity in research with young children' in P. Christensen and A. James (eds) *Research with Children: Perspectives and Practices* (2nd edn), London: Routledge.

Cook, T. and Hess, E. (2007) 'What the camera sees and from whose perspective? Fun methodologies for engaging children in enlightening adults', *Childhood*, 14(1), 29–46.

Corby, B. (2000) *Child Abuse: Towards a Knowledge Base*, Maidenhead: Open University Press.

Corby, B., Doig, A. and Roberts, V. (1998) 'Inquiries into child abuse', *Journal of Social Welfare and Family Law*, 20(4), 377–95.

Cousins, W., Monteith, M., Larkin, E. and Percy, A. (2003) *The Care Careers of Younger Looked After Children: Findings from the Multiple Placement Project*, Belfast: Institute of Child Care Research, University of Belfast.

Crompton, M. (1980) *Respecting Children: Social Work with Young People*, London: Edward Arnold Publishers.

Curtis, M. (1946) *Report of the Care of Children Committee*, Cmd 6922, London: His Majesty's Stationery Office.

Danby, S. and Farrell, A. (2004) 'Accounting for young children's competence in educational research: new perspectives on research ethics', *The Australian Educational Researcher*, 31(3), 35–49.

Darbyshire, P., MacDougall, C. and Schiller, W. (2005) 'Multiple methods in qualitative research with children: more insight or just more?', *Qualitative Research*, 5(4), 417–36.

Davie, R., Upton, G. and Varma, V. (eds) (1996) *The Voice of the Child: A Handbook for Professionals*, London: Falmer Press.

Department for Children, Schools and Families (DCSF) (2007) *The Children's Plan: Building Brighter Futures*, London: The Stationery Office.

—— (2008a) *Care Matters: Time to Deliver for Children in Care*, London: HM Government/ Association of Directors of Children's Services/Local Government Association.

—— (2008b) *Piloting the Social Work Practice Model: A Prospectus*, Nottingham: Department for Children, Schools and Families.

—— (2009a) *The Protection of Children in England: Action Plan. The Government's Response to Lord Laming*, Cm 7589, London: The Stationery Office.

—— (2009b) *Children Looked After in England (Including Adoption and Care Leavers) Year Ending 31 March 2009*, London: Department for Children, Schools and Families.

—— (2009c) *Social Work Task Force: Building a Safe, Confident Future; The Final Report of the Social Work Task Force, November 2009*, London: Department for Children, Schools and Families.

—— (2009d) *Social Work Task Force: First Report of the Social Work Task Force*, London: Department for Children, Schools and Families.

—— (2010a) *Building a Safe and Confident Future: Implementing the Recommendations of the Social Work Task Force*, London: Department for Children, Schools and Families.

—— (2010b) *Working Together to Safeguard Children: A Guide to Inter-Agency Working to Safeguard and Promote the Welfare of Children*, Nottingham: Department for Children, Schools and Families.

—— (2010c) *The Children Act 1989 Guidance and Regulations. Volume 2: Care Planning, Placement and Case Review*, London: Department for Children, Schools and Families.

Department for Children, Schools and Families (DCSF) Children's Rights and Participation Team (2010) *The United Nations Convention on the Rights of the Child: How Legislation Underpins Implementation in England; Further Information for the Joint Committee on Human Rights*, London: Department for Children, Schools and Families.

Department for Education and Skills (DfES) (2004a) *Common Assessment Framework*, London: The Stationery Office.

—— (2004b) *Every Child Matters: Next Steps*, Nottingham: DfES Publications.

—— (2005) *Common Core of Skills and Knowledge for the Children's Workforce*, London: HM Government.

—— (2006) *Care Matters: Transforming the Lives of Children and Young People in Care*, London: HMSO.

—— (2007) *Care Matters: Consultation Responses*, London: HMSO.

Department for Education and Skills and National Children's Bureau (DfES/NCB) (2006) *Communicating with Children: A Two-Way Process*, London: Department for Education and Skills and National Children's Bureau.

Department of Health (DH) (1998a) *Quality Protects: Framework for Action*, London: HMSO.

—— (1998b) *Quality Protects: Transforming Children's Services*, London: Department of Health.

—— (1998c) *Modernising Social Services: Promoting Independence, Improving Protection, Raising Standards*, London: The Stationery Office.

—— (1999a) *The Quality Protects Programme: Transforming Children's Services 2000/2001*, London: Department of Health.

—— (1999b) *The Government Objectives for Children's Social Services*. London: Department of Health.

Department of Health (DH) and Department for Children, Schools and Families (DCSF) (2009) *Facing up to the Task: The Interim Report of the Social Work Task Force; July 2009*, London: Department of Health and Department for Children, Schools and Families.

Department of Health (DH), Department for Education and Employment and Home Office (2000) *Framework for the Assessment of Children in Need and their Families*, London: The Stationery Office.

—— (2002) *Listening, Hearing and Responding: Core Principles for the Involvement of Children*, London: The Stationery Office.

Department of Health and Social Security (DHSS) (1974) *Report of the Committee of Inquiry into the Care and Supervision Provided in Relation to Maria Colwell*, London: HMSO.

—— (1982) *Child Abuse: A Study of Inquiry Reports 1973–1981*, London: HMSO.

—— (1988) *Report of the Inquiry into Child Abuse in Cleveland*, London: HMSO.

Department of Health, Social Services and Public Safety Northern Ireland (DHSSPSNI) (2003) *Co-operating to Safeguard Children*, Belfast: Department of Health, Social Services and Public Safety Northern Ireland.

—— (2007) *Care Matters in Northern Ireland: Building a Bridge to a Better Future*, Belfast: Department of Health, Social Services and Public Safety Northern Ireland.

—— (2008) *Understanding the Needs of Children in Northern Ireland (UNOCINI)*, Belfast: Department of Health, Social Services and Public Safety Northern Ireland.

—— (2010) *Children Order Statistical Bulletin 2009*, Belfast: Department of Health, Social Services and Public Safety Northern Ireland.

Dingwall, R., Eekalaar, J. and Murray, T. (1983) *The Protection of Children: State, Intervention and Family Life*, Oxford: Blackwell.

Dockett, S. and Perry, B. (2007) 'Trusting children's accounts in research', *Journal of Early Childhood Research*, 5(47), 47–63.

Einarsdottir, J., Dockett, S. and Perry, B. (2009) 'Making meaning: children's perspectives expressed through drawings', *Early Child Development and Care*, 179(2), 217–32.

Fasoli, L. (2003) 'Reading photographs of young children: looking at practices', *Contemporary Issues in Early Childhood*, 4(1), 32–47.

Ferguson, H. (2005) 'Working with violence, the emotions and the psycho-social dynamics of child protection: reflections on the Victoria Climbié case', *Social Work Education*, 24(7), 781–95.

Fletcher, B. (1993) *Not Just a Name: The Views of Young People in Residential and Foster Care*, London: National Consumer Council.

Flewitt, R. (2005) 'Conducting research with young children: some ethical considerations', *Early Child Development and Care*, 175(6), 553–65.

Garrett, P. M. (2008) 'Social work practices: silences and elisions in the plan to "transform" the lives of children "looked after" in England', *Child and Family Social Work*, 13(3), 311–18.

General Social Care Council (GSCC), Commission for Social Care Inspection, Children's Development Workforce Council and Social Care Institute for Excellence and Skills for Care (2008) *Social Work at its Best: A Statement of Social Work Roles and Tasks for the 21st Century*, London: General Social Care Council.

Gilligan, P. and Manby, M. (2008) 'The Common Assessment Framework: does the reality match the rhetoric?', *Child and Family Social Work*, 3(2), 177–87.

Gilligan, R. (2001) *Promoting Resilience: A Resource Guide on Working with Children in the Care System*, London: BAAF.

Green, D. (2007) 'Risk and social work practice', *Australian Social Work*, 60(4), 395–409.

Greig, A., Minnis, H., Millward, R., Sinclair, C., Kennedy, E., Towlson, K., Reid, W. and Hill, J. (2008) 'Relationships and learning: a review and investigation of narrative coherence in looked-after children in primary school', *Educational Psychology in Practice*, 24(1), 13–27.

Gupta, A. and Blewitt, J. (2007) 'Change for children? Challenges and opportunities for the children's social work workforce', *Child and Family Social Work*, 12, 172–81.

Haringey Local Safeguarding Children Board (LSCB) (2009) *Serious Case Review: Baby Peter*, Haringey: Haringey Local Safeguarding Children Board.

Hill, M. (1997) 'Research review: participatory research with children', *Child and Family Social Work*, 2, 171–83.

—— (2006) 'Children's voices on ways of having a voice', *Childhood*, 13(1), 69–89.

HM Government (2006) *Working Together to Safeguard Children: A Guide to Inter-Agency*

Working to Safeguard and Promote the Welfare of Children, London: The Stationery Office.

—— (2009) *The Protection of Children in England: Action Plan. The Government's Response to Lord Laming*, London: The Stationery Office.

HM Treasury (2003) *Every Child Matters*, London: The Stationery Office.

Holland, S. (2004) *Child and Family Assessment in Social Work Practice*, London: Sage.

Holmes, L., McDermid, S., Jones, S. and Ward, H. (2009) *How Social Workers Spend Their Time: An Analysis of the Key Issues that Impact on Practice Pre- and Post Implementation of the Integrated Children's System*, London: Department for Children, Schools and Families.

Home Department (1945) *Report by Sir Walter Monckton KCMG, KCVO, MC, KC on the Circumstances Which Led to the Boarding Out of Dennis and Terence O'Neill at Bank Farm, Ministerley and the Steps Taken to Supervise their Welfare*, Cmd 6636, London: His Majesty's Stationery Office.

Home Department, Ministry of Health, Ministry of Education (1946) *Report of the Care Of Children Committee*, Cmd 6922, London: His Majesty's Stationery Office.

Horwath, J. (2009) *The Child's World: The Comprehensive Guide to Assessing Children in Need* (2nd edn), London: Jessica Kingsley Publishers.

House of Commons Children, Schools and Families Select Committee (HC CSF) (2009) *Training of Children and Families Social Workers: Seventh Report of Session 2008–2009, Volume 1 (HC527–1)*, London: The Stationery Office.

Houston, S. and Knox, S. (2004) 'Exploring workforce retention in child and family social work: critical social theory, social pedagogy and action research', *Social Work and Social Sciences Review*, 11(2), 36–53.

Howe, D. (2008) *The Emotionally Intelligent Social Worker*, Basingstoke: Palgrave Macmillan.

Human Rights Act (1998) Available online: www.opsi.gov.uk/ACTS/acts1998/ukpga_19980042_en_1

James, A. and Prout, A. (eds) (1997) *Constructing and Reconstructing Childhood*, London: Falmer Press.

Jenks, C. (ed.) (1982) *The Sociology of Childhood: Essential Readings*, London: Batsford Academic and Educational.

Jones, D. P. H. (2003) *Communicating with Vulnerable Children: A Guide for Practitioners*, London: Gaskell.

Kilkelly, U., Kilpatrick, R., Lundy, L., Moore, L., Scraton, P., Davey, C., Dwyer, C. and McAlister, S. (2004) *Children's Rights in Northern Ireland*, Belfast: Northern Ireland Commissioner for Children and Young People.

Kirby, P., Lanyon, C., Kronin, K. and Sinclair, R. (2003) *Building a Culture of Participation: Involving Children and Young People in Policy, Service Planning, Delivery and Evaluation*. London: National Children's Bureau/Department for Education and Skills.

Koprowska, J. (2008) *Communication and Interpersonal Skills in Social Work* (2nd edn), Exeter: Learning Matters.

Kortesluoma, R. L., Hentinen, M. and Nikkonen, M. (2003) 'Conducting a qualitative child interview: methodological considerations', *Journal of Advanced Nursing*, 42(5), 434–41.

Laming, Lord H. (2003) *The Victoria Climbié Inquiry*, London: The Stationery Office.

—— (2008) 'Child protection plans failing', Available online: http://news.bbc.co.uk/1/hi/programmes/file_on_4/7200217.stm

—— (2009) *The Protection of Children in England: A Progress Report*, London: The Stationery Office.

Lansdown, G. (2005a) *Can You Hear Me? The Right of Young Children to Participate in Decisions Affecting Them*, The Hague: Bernard Van Leer Foundation.

—— (2005b) *The Evolving Capacities of Children: Implications for the Exercise of Rights*, Florence: UNICEF Innocenti Research Centre.

Larsson, A. and Lamb, M. E. (2009) 'Making the most of information-gathering interviews with children', *Infant and Child Development*, 18, 1–16

Le Grand, J. (2007) *Consistent Care Matters: Exploring the Potential of Social Work Practices*, London: Department for Education and Skills.

Leeson, C. (2007) 'My life in care: experiences of non-participation in decision-making processes', *Child and Family Social Work*, 12, 268–77.

—— (2009) 'The involvement of looked-after children in making decisions about their present and future care needs', PhD thesis, University of Plymouth: unpublished.

Lefevre, M. (2008) 'Communicating and engaging with children and young people in care through play and the creative arts', in B. Luckock and M. Lefevre (eds) *Direct Work: Social Work with Children and Young People in Care*, London: British Association for Adoption and Fostering.

—— (2010) *Communicating with Children and Young People: Making a Difference*, London: Policy Press.

Lefevre, M., Tanner, K. and Luckock, B. (2008) 'Developing social work students' communication skills with children and young people: a model for the qualifying level curriculum', *Child and Family Social Work*, 13, 166–76.

Levy, A. and Kahan, B. (1991) *The Pindown Experience and the Protection of Children*, Stafford: Staffordshire County Council.

London Borough of Brent (1985) *A Child in Trust: The Report of the Panel of Inquiry into the Circumstances Surrounding the Death of Jasmine Beckford*, London: London Borough of Brent.

London Borough of Greenwich (1987) *A Child in Mind: Report of the Commission of Inquiry into the Circumstances Surrounding the Death of Kimberley Carlisle*, London: London Borough of Greenwich.

London Borough of Lambeth (1987) *Whose Child? The Report of the Public Inquiry into the Death of Tyra Henry*, London: London Borough of Lambeth.

Luckock, B. and Lefevre, M. (eds) (2008) *Direct Work: Social Work with Children and Young People in Care*, London: British Association for Adoption and Fostering.

Luckock, B., Lefevre, M. and Tanner, K. (2007) 'Teaching and learning communication with children and young people: developing the qualifying social work curriculum in a changing policy context', *Child and Family Social Work*, 12(2), 192–201.

Luckock, B., Stevens, P. and Young, J. (2008) 'Living through the experience: the social worker as trusted ally and champion of young people in care', in B. Luckock and M. Lefevre (eds) *Direct Work: Social Work with Children and Young People in Care*, London: British Association for Adoption and Fostering.

Lynes, D. and Goddard, J. (1995) *The View from the Front: The User View of Child Care in Norfolk*, Norwich: Norfolk In-Care Group, Norfolk County Council.

McLeod, A. (2001) 'Listening but not hearing: barriers to effective communication between children in public care and their social workers', PhD thesis, University of Lancaster.

—— (2006) 'Respect or empowerment? Alternative understandings of "listening" in childcare social work', *Adoption and Fostering*, 30(4), 43–52.

—— (2007) 'Whose agenda? Issues of power and relationship when listening to looked-after young people', *Child and Family Social Work*, 12(3), 278–86.

—— (2008a) '"A friend and an equal": do young people in care seek the impossible from their social workers?', *British Journal Social Work*, Advance Access, 40(3), 772–88.

—— (2008b) *Listening to Children: A Practitioner's Guide*, London: Jessica Kingsley Publishers.

MacNaughton, G. (2003) 'Eclipsing voice in research with young children', *Australian Journal of Early Childhood*, 28(1), 36–43.

McSherry, D., Larking, E. and Iwaniec, D. (2006) 'Care proceedings: exploring the relationship between case duration and achieving permanency for the child', *British Journal of Social Work*, 36, 901–19.

Marchant, R. (2008) 'Working with disabled children who are looked after' in B. Luckock and M. Lefevre (eds) *Direct Work: Social Work with Children and Young People in Care*, London: BAAF.

Masson, J., Pearce, J., Bader, K., Joyner, O., Marsden, J. and Westlake, D. (2008) *Ministry of Justice Research Series 4/08: Care Profiling Study*, London: Ministry of Justice.

Milner, P. and Carolin, B. (1999/2000) *Time to Listen to Children: Personal and Professional Communication*, London: Routledge.

Monteith, M. and Cousins, W. (2003) 'The importance of stability in the lives of looked after children: a study of under fives in Northern Ireland', *Child Care in Practice*, 9(1), 62–71.

Morgan, R. (2006) *About Social Workers: A Children's Views Report*, Newcastle Upon Tyne: Commission for Social Care Inspection.

Morrison, T. (2007) 'Emotional intelligence, emotion and social work: context, characteristics, complications and contribution', *British Journal of Social Work*, 37, 245–63.

Munro, E. (2001) 'Empowering looked after children', *Child and Family Social Work*, 6(2), 129–38.

Munro, E. R. and Ward, H. (2008) 'Balancing parents' and very young children's rights in care proceedings: decision-making in the context of the Human Rights Act 1998', *Child and Family Social Work*, 13, 227–34.

National Children's Bureau (NCB) (2004) *Listening as a Way of Life*, London: National Children's Bureau.

—— (2006) 'Communicating with children during assessment', Available online: www.ncb.org. uk/resources/free_resources/communicating_with_children.aspx

Northern Ireland Commissioner for Children and Young People (NICCY) (2006) *Review of Children and Young People's Participation in the Care Planning Process*, Belfast: Northern Ireland Commissioner for Children and Young People.

O'Kane, C. (2008) 'The development of participatory techniques: facilitating children's views about decisions affecting them' in P. Christensen and A. James (eds) *Research with Children: Perspectives and Practices*, London: Routledge.

O'Neill, K. (2008) *Getting it Right for Children: A Practitioners' Guide to Children's Rights*, London: Save the Children UK.

O'Neill, T. (2010) *Someone to Love Us: The Shocking True Story of Two Brothers Fostered into Brutality and Neglect*, London: Harper Element.

Packman, J., Randall, J. and Jacques, N. (1986) *Who Needs Care? Social Work Decisions about Children*, Oxford: Basil Blackwell.

Page, R. and Clark, G. A. (eds) (1977) *Who Cares? Young People in Care Speak Out*, London: National Children's Bureau.

Parton, N. (2004) 'From Maria Colwell to Victoria Climbié: reflections on public inquiries into child abuse a generation apart', *Child Abuse Review*, 30, 80–94.

—— (2006) *Safeguarding Childhood: Early Intervention and Surveillance in a Late Modern Society*, Basingstoke: Palgrave Macmillan.

Philpot, T. (2000) Barbara Kahan: childcare pioneer whose 'pindown' scandal report prompted residential care reform, Available online: www.guardian.co.uk/news/2000/aug/09/guardianobituaries2

Pithouse, A. (2006) 'A common assessment for children in need? Mixed messages from a pilot study in Wales', *Child Care in Practice*, 12(3), 199–217.

Pithouse, A., Hall, C., Peckover, S. and White, S. (2009) 'A tale of two CAFs: the impact of the electronic Common Assessment Framework', *British Journal of Social Work*, 39(4), 599–612.

Prout A. and James, A. (1997) 'A new paradigm for the sociology of childhood? Provenance, promise and problems' in A. James and A. Prout (eds) *Constructing and Reconstructing Childhood*, London: Falmer Press.

Punch, S. (2002a) 'Interviewing strategies with young people: the "secret box", stimulus material and task-based activities', *Children and Society*, 16, 45–56.

—— (2002b) 'Research with children: the same or different from research with adults?', *Childhood*, 9(3), 321–41.

—— (2007) '"I felt they were ganging up on me": interviewing siblings at home', *Children's Geographies*, 5(3), 219–34.

Ruch, G. (2010a) 'The contemporary context of relationship-based practice', in G. Ruch, D. Turney and A. Ward (eds) *Relationship-Based Social Work: Getting to the Heart of Practice*, London: Jessica Kingsley Publishers.

—— (2010b) 'Theoretical frameworks informing relationship-based practice,' in G. Ruch, D. Turney and A. Ward (eds) *Relationship-Based Social Work: Getting to the Heart of Practice*, London: Jessica Kingsley Publishers.

Ruch, G., Turney, D. and Ward, A. (2010) *Relationship Based Social Work: Getting to the Heart of Practice*, London: Jessica Kingsley Publishers.

Schofield, G. (2005) 'The voice of the child in family placement decision making: a developmental model', *Adoption and Fostering*, 19(1), 29–44.

Scottish Alliance for Children's Rights (SACR) (2009) *Improving the Lives of Children in Scotland: Are We There Yet? Findings from National Seminars January-February 2009*, Glasgow: ACR.

Scottish Executive (2004a) *Protecting Children and Young People: The Charter*, Edinburgh: Scottish Executive.

—— (2004b) *Protecting Children and Young People: Framework for Standards*, Edinburgh: Scottish Executive.

—— (2005) *Summary Report of the 21st Century Social Work Review*, Edinburgh: Scottish Executive.

Scottish Government (2008) *Guide to Getting it Right for Every Child*, Available online: www. scotland.gov.uk/Publications/2008/09/22091734/0

—— (2010) *Statistics Publication Notice: Health and Care Series; Children Looked After Statistics 2008–2009*, Edinburgh: Scottish Government.

Sempik, J., Ward, H. and Darker, I. (2008) 'Emotional and behavioural difficulties of children and young people at entry into care', *Clinical Child Psychology and Psychiatry*, 13(2), 221–33.

Sinclair, R. (1984) *Decision-Making in Statutory Reviews on Children in Care*, Aldershot: Gower.

—— (2004) 'Participation in practice: making it meaningful, effective and sustainable', *Children and Society*, 18(2), 106–18.

Social Care Institute of Excellence (SCIE)(2010) 'Communication skills', Available online: www. scie.org.uk/publications/elearning/cs/index.asp

Social Work Task Force (SWTF) (2009a) *Building a Safe, Confident Future: The Final Report of the Social Work Task Force*, London: Department of Children, Schools and Families.

—— (2009b) *First Report of the Social Work Task Force*, London: Department of Children, Schools and Families.

Stanley, J. and Goddard, C. (1997) 'Failures in child protection: a case study', *Child Abuse Review*, 6, 46–54.

—— (2002) *In the Firing Line: Violence and Power in Child Protection Work*, Chichester: John Wiley & Sons.

Statham, J., Cameron, C. and Mooney, A. (2006) *The Tasks and Roles of Social Workers: A Focused Overview of Research Evidence*, London: Thomas Coram Research Unit.

Stevenson, O. (1986) 'Guest editorial on the Jasmine Beckford inquiry', *British Journal Social Work*, 16, 501–10.

Taylor, C. (2004) 'Underpinning knowledge for childcare practice: reconsidering child development theory', *Child and Family Social Work*, 9, 225–35.

Thomas, N. and O'Kane, C. (1998) *Children and Decision-Making: A Summary Report*, Swansea: International Centre for Childhood Studies, University of Wales.

—— (1999) 'Children's participation in reviews and planning meetings when they are "looked after" in middle childhood', *Child and Family Social Work*, 4, 221–30.

Trevithick, P. (2005) *Social Work Skills: A Practice Handbook* (2nd edn), Maidenhead: Open University Press.

Turney, D. J. (2008) 'The power of the gaze: observation and its role in direct practice with children in care', in B. Luckock and M. Lefevre (eds), *Direct Work with Children and Young People: A Guide to Social Work Practice in Fostering, Adoption and Residential Care*, London: BAAF, pp. 115–29.

Turney, D., Ward, A. and Ruch, G. (2010) 'Conclusion' in in G. Ruch, D. Turney and A. Ward (eds) *Relationship-Based Social Work: Getting to the Heart of Practice*, London: Jessica Kingsley Publishers.

United Nations (UN) (1989) *Convention on the Rights of the Child*, Geneva: United Nations.

—— (2003) *General Comment No. 5: General Measures of Implementation for the Convention on the Rights of the Child*, Geneva: United Nations.

—— (2005) *General Comment No. 7: Implementing Child Rights in Early Childhood*, Geneva: United Nations.

—— (2007) *General Comment No. 7: The Rights of Children with Disabilities*, Geneva: United Nations.

—— (2008) *Concluding Observations: United Kingdom of Great Britain and Northern Ireland*, Geneva: United Nations.

—— (2009) *General Comment No. 12: The Right of the Child to be Heard*, Geneva: United Nations.

Utting, W. (1991) *Children in the Public Care: A Review of Residential Child Care*, London: HMSO.

—— (1997) *People like Us: The Report of the Review of Safeguards for Children Living Away from Home*, London: Department of Health/Welsh Office.

Vernon, J. and Fruin, D. (1986) *In Care: A Study of Social Work Decision Making*, London: National Children's Bureau.

Voice (2010) *Blueprint in Practice: Partnership Projects*, London: Voice.

Voice for the Child in Care/National Children's Bureau (VCC/NCB) (2004) *Start with the Child: Stay with the Child*, London: Voice for the Child in Care/National Children's Bureau.

Ward, A. (2010a) 'The use of self in relationship-based practice', in G. Ruch, D. Turney and A. Ward (eds) *Relationship-Based Social Work: Getting to the Heart of Practice*, London: Jessica Kingsley Publishers.

—— (2010b) 'The learning relationship: learning and development for relationship-based practice', in G. Ruch, D. Turney and A. Ward (eds) *Relationship-Based Social Work: Getting to the Heart of Practice*, London: Jessica Kingsley Publishers.

Ward, H. (2009) 'Patterns of instability: moves within the care system, their reasons, contexts and consequences', *Children and Youth Services Review*, 31(10), 1113–18.

Ward, H., Munro, E. and Dearden, C. (2006) *Babies and Young Children in Care: Life Pathways, Decision-Making and Practice*, London: Jessica Kingsley Publishers.

Waterhouse, R., Clough, M. and Le Fleming, M. J. (2000) *Lost in Care: Report of the Tribunal of Inquiry into the Abuse of Children in Care in the Former County Council Areas of Gwynedd and Clwyd since 1974*, London: The Stationery Office.

Watson, D. and West, J. (2006) *Social Work Process and Practice: Approaches, Knowledge and Skills*, Basingstoke: Palgrave Macmillan. Webb, S. (2006) *Social Work in a Risk Society*, New York: Palgrave Macmillan.

Welbourne, P. (2002) 'Culture, children's rights and child protection', *Child Abuse Review*, 11(6), 345–58.

Welsh Assembly Government (2009) *Adoptions, Outcomes and Placements for Children Looked*

After by Local Authorities: Year Ending 31 March 2009, Cardiff: Health Statistics and Analysis Unit.

What Makes the Difference project (WMTD) (2007) *Care Matters: WMTD Response*, London: What Makes the Difference? Project.

Wilson, K., Ruch, G., Lymbery, M. and Cooper, A. (2008) *Social Work: An Introduction to Contemporary Practice*, Edinburgh: Pearson Education.

Winter, K. (2006) 'Widening our knowledge concerning young looked after children: the case for research using sociological models of childhood', *Child and Family Social Work*, 11, 55–64.

—— (2009) 'Relationships matter: the problems and prospects for social workers' relationships with young children in care', *Child and Family Social Work*, 14(4), 450–60.

—— (2010) 'The perspectives of young children in care about their circumstances and implications for social work practice', *Child and Family Social Work*, 15, 186–95.

Winter, K. and Cohen, O. (2005) 'Identity issues for looked after children with no knowledge of their origins: implications for research and practice', *Adoption and Fostering*, 29(2), 44–52.

Winter, K. and Connolly, P. (2005) 'A small scale study of the relationship between measures of deprivation and child care referrals', *British Journal of Social Work*, 35(6), 937–52.

Index

access: to information 22, 29, 32, 58, 72, 77, 97, 102, 138, 140; to services 58, 63, 96, 137, 140, 144
accountability 17, 58, 72–3, 100, 109, 138–9, 147–9
Adoption and Children Act 2002 32
age-related factors 11, 13, 20, 25–6, 31–2, 42, 47–9, 51, 53–4, 58, 62, 64–5, 67–8, 70–2, 97, 100–1, 104, 138, 142–3, 146–7
alcohol 75, 111, 120, 128
anxiety 12, 29, 41–3, 45, 51, 63, 80, 120
assessment 13, 16, 19–20, 30–2, 36, 39, 41–3, 48, 53, 61, 63, 66, 68–9, 75, 86, 130, 136–8, 142, 148–9
assumptions by social workers 8, 12, 16, 47–9, 56, 58, 63–4, 66, 68, 71, 89, 98, 101, 116, 138, 147, 150 see also habitus
attachment 27–8
attitude of social workers 16, 24, 54, 68, 72, 81, 134, 144
audit tool 57, 134, 146–9

'Baby P' see Connelly, Peter
barriers 4, 37–57, 61, 101, 134, 137, 147–8, 150
Beckford, Jasmine 2, 14–16, 64–5, 69
behaviour 23, 26–8, 35, 42, 45, 54, 66, 69, 81, 88–90, 102, 128, 136
belonging, sense of 29
best interests of child 17, 43, 59, 62, 64–6, 73, 127, 138, 142–3, 146
Blom-Cooper, Louis 14
Blueprint Project 21–2, 35
body language 65, 72, 81, 90, 98–9, 102, 140
boundaries 4, 35, 63, 97, 102–3, 107, 118, 126–7, 132, 139–40; testing 90
Bourdieu, Pierre 38, 103
Bronfenbrenner, Urie 69
bureaucracy 2, 7, 40–1, 57
Butler-Sloss, Baroness Elizabeth 16–17

CAF (Common Assessment Framework) 30–1, 41, 43, 61
capacity of children see competence of children
Care Matters 21–2, 28, 61, 67
Carlisle, Kimberley 2, 14
caseload 9–11, 19, 21, 28, 37, 41, 51–2, 145, 147
child: abuse 7, 14, 16, 58, 62, 66–7, 86, 136, 150 see also neglect of child; protection 1–2, 14, 19, 30, 50, 68, 98–9, 110, 145
child protection register 1, 14, 26
Childcare Act 2006 60
children: in care 3, 13, 16, 21–2, 26–30, 32, 34–7, 41, 44–5, 48, 51–2, 54–5, 61, 66, 75, 82, 90, 106, 111, 118, 120, 140, 149; in need 20, 26, 30–2, 41, 61, 68; at risk 15, 20, 26, 30–1, 36, 41, 61, 63
Children Act 1948 11
Children Act 1975 13, 17
Children Act 1989 17, 22, 32, 60
Children Act 2004 20, 60–1
Children (Leaving Care) Act 2000 32
Children (Scotland) Act 1995 32, 60
Children (Northern Ireland) Order 1995 32, 60
children's: commissioner 60; officers 11; rights commissioners 60
Children's Rights Alliance for England 61
Children's Workforce Development Council 20–1, 34, 50
choice 4, 104; of child 27, 33, 45, 48, 60, 64, 77–9, 81, 88, 90–1, 95, 97–9, 101, 106–7, 110, 113, 122, 129–30, 132, 138, 140, 144, 147
Cleveland Inquiry 1988 16–17
Climbié, Victoria 2, 7, 18–19, 27, 46, 57, 63, 66–7
Colwell, Maria 2, 11, 13, 64–6, 145
competence of children 3–4, 33, 47–9, 53–4, 56, 64–5, 67–8, 70–2, 76, 82, 89–90, 98,